Praise for *My Turn*

"A deeply inspiring narrative of one family and their journey of living and loving fully throughout generations of cancer diagnoses. Beautifully written, *My Turn on the Couch* is a treasure of lessons for all of us on how to live an authentic life filled with joy, vitality and intimacy regardless of prognosis. The Alimenti family has given us all a gift by sharing their story and truly being an exemplar of resilience."

—Susan Bauer-Wu, PhD, RN, FAAN, President of the Mind & Life
Institute and author of *Leaves Falling Gently*

"*My Turn on the Couch* is a hopeful, inspiring work of beauty. Carol's voice—strong, faithful, loving, and kind—comes alive on the pages of this book as she describes her family's and her own cancer journey. Despite the many seemingly insurmountable battles she faced, Carol never lost her faith, nor her optimism. Her words are a powerful reminder to find humor in life and to love and appreciate your body, your family, your health, and your life, for tomorrow is not promised."

—Rachael Palm, Communications Coordinator, Hospice of the Piedmont

"Although *My Turn on the Couch* is about a family riddled with cancer, it's not a story about death. It's about life, and the remarkable life of Carol Alimenti and her family.

Their navigation through one of the most treacherous of enemies is a life lesson for us all. Carol's son and mother were already battling the disease when Carol was diagnosed with a rare sarcoma. She lived seven years when she was given only fifteen months. This book is her story of maneuvering through those years, not just surviving, but living, loving and laughing while struggling with enormous pain, chemo, radiation and numerous surgeries.

My Turn on the Couch doesn't back away from everything Carol goes through, but it embraces how she goes through it. With diet, rest, yoga, restorative therapy, music, art, reading, movies, travel, determination, breathing right and, above all, humor and faith, Carol, her husband Tony, her son Chris and daughter Darcy show us how to hug each day. You will feel less likely to complain about the minutia most of us find irritating, and instead relish even the smallest miracles of the everyday."

—Carol Donsky Newell, author of *Blue Lewis and Sasha the Great*,
Flight of the Kiwi and *A Perfect Spring Day*. She is an award-winning
journalist, film critic and teacher.

My Turn on the Couch

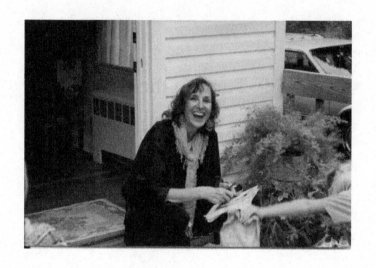

My Turn on the Couch:
Our Cancer Journey

by Carol Alimenti
Tony Alimenti
Christopher Alimenti
and Darcy Alimenti

BELLE ISLE BOOKS
www.belleislebooks.com

ISBN: 978-1-9399309-3-4

Library of Congress Control Number: 2017946878

Printed in the United States

Published by

BELLE ISLE BOOKS
www.belleislebooks.com

This book is dedicated to Anna Lemma, "Nana," whose beauty and grace, despite hardships, always prevailed; and to all of those whose lives have been touched by cancer.

TABLE OF CONTENTS

"Life should not be a journey to the grave with the intention of arriving safely in a pretty and well-preserved body, but rather to skid in broadside in a cloud of smoke, thoroughly used up, totally worn out, and loudly proclaiming, 'Wow! What a RIDE!'"

—Hunter S. Thompson

Prologue

Psalm 91:4 He will cover you with His feathers, and under His wings you will find refuge.

When I was a child, my parents' bedroom came to symbolize a place of honor: the throne of respite and healing. If I suffered from any ailment, from a mere runny nose to a debilitating cough, I comfortably idled away the daytime hours curled up on my parents' oversized mattress. My mother would fuss over me like a protective, doting mother hen. The bedside table would mysteriously transform into an arsenal of soothing items from tissues to a bedside bell. Yes—a bell, which I was to ring whenever I, queen for the day, needed anything from pillow fluffing to the next dose of magic elixir. It was my princess time, when I received the royal treatment, the spa offering, the "Full Monty"!

Alas, I was not, however, the only family member to receive this royal protocol. My (in my mind's eye, undeserving) siblings also got their turns on the majestic mattress. Lounging in our parents' bed was a huge treat, because my folks had a strict taboo against kids climbing into their bed at night. When awakened by frightening dreams, we were gently soothed, then ushered back to our respective beds, like sheep being herded back into their corral. Receiving a turn on the coveted special recuperating vessel was especially exciting for me because my younger sister, due to a childhood illness, was a real bed hog. In stark contrast, I was the family's prized foal: "healthy as a horse."

So it was only natural that when I became a mom, I would initiate a similar routine for an ailing family member. Instead of

i

the bed, I chose the couch. Why the couch, you might ask? This decision, as I reflect back, probably had more to do with our home's floor plan than anything else. In both scenarios, the sick were closest to the hub of activity: the kitchen. Hence, the title of this book, *My Turn on the Couch*, was born from a combination of childhood memories and my aging mother claiming the couch as her rightful domain after being diagnosed with cancer for the third time. I also followed my mother's lead and positioned a snack table at the side of the couch and, as my mother had done, filled it with all the necessary tools and paraphernalia to aid in the healing process.

As a mom, I never imagined that our couch would be called upon to function as a place of healing respite so often, or that so many family members would rotate through it. This is our story—my family's intimate tale of our journey with illness, primarily the big "C," cancer. It is a story that outlines the bumps in our lives and the subsequent role our couch has played in the journey of healing—the healing of mind, body and soul.

"Sometimes you will never know the value of a moment until it becomes a memory."

—Dr. Seuss

Part I
Our Life Unraveled

Chapter 1
Why?

Isaiah 55:9   As the heavens are higher than the earth, so are My ways higher than your ways, and My thoughts than your thoughts.

September, the month my son was born, has arrived. Autumn, my favorite season, is upon us. Summer is quickly fading; the dog days and oppressive heat are abating. This time of year always brings with it mixed feelings: a readiness for the kids to jump back into the school routine, but grief for the loss of the lazy days summer affords. Schools are prepared and ready for the onslaught of those eager and those more reluctant students to fill their halls. Evenings are cooling off, while the leaves are beginning to ignite our world with a spectacle of color, much like a July 4th fireworks display. Life feels good.

My eldest, Chris, is entering his second year of high school. Having spent the summer contentedly as a camp counselor in the Shenandoah Mountains of Virginia, he returned home with an air of confidence, his manhood emerging into his being like a gathering storm. He shocked us all with a growth spurt of five inches. A summer of being on his own—no nagging parents, no lawn to mow, no bedroom to clean; simply camping, swimming, and boating—outfitted him with a euphoric, adolescent high much like a cloud soaring on the edge of the horizon. Little did we know that a different, unfamiliar reality would soon decimate his newly found world like an arrow to the heart, a pervasive darkness.

Shortly after his arrival home from "camp utopia," he began

reluctantly training for a four-miler with his dad. Chris was not necessarily an athletic kid and running was not his forte, but this race was not about athletic prowess but more about a dad desiring a father–son bonding experience. When Chris, a normally noncomplaining sort, started walking with difficulty and mentioning in a nonchalant fashion that his legs were hurting, no great alarms sounded. We naturally assumed it was all related to the prerace training.

As Chris's legs trembled with increasingly agonizing pain, my anxiety rose, and I reached out to my "all-knowing" mother. I reported the leg pain Chris was experiencing and she confidently, but with a sense of urgency, instructed me to have a doctor examine him for rheumatoid arthritis, ASAP. She had suffered with leg pain as a youth, and rheumatoid arthritis had been the culprit. So, without hesitation, I made an appointment; and because I stressed the critical nature of the visit, we were at the doctor's office within days.

The visit assured us that Chris's pain was indeed NOT rheumatoid arthritis. This would cause redness and swelling of the joints, which Chris did not have. The doctor felt that Chris's huge growth spurt and increased physical activity may have been the culprits. Somewhat comforted, but still leery and uncertain, we headed back home. I procured muscle ointments for Chris to apply regularly, and continually urged him to soak his weary limbs in our hot tub. Despite the remedies, his pain only worsened, resulting in a second visit to the doctor. We were once again reassured that it was only the product of overstressed muscles, but to please me, he would refer us to an orthopedic. The word "orthopedic" brought back humbling memories of the insecure mother that I had been, dragging my six-year-old son to the doctor so he could inform me that the protruding bones on Chris's back were due to his extremely slight build, and not a bone deformity as I had anxiously imagined. Now, should I risk running him yet again to another specialist, only to soothe my neurotic-mother syndrome? Doubts raced through my mind. Was I manufacturing diseases for my children? Was I being overly dramatic? Why was I always anticipating the worst? I decided to bring to a halt the musings of my overactive brain and play it cool, taking on the wait-and-see philosophy.

As October began to fade away, as the days grew shorter and the evenings required an extra layer of clothing, new symptoms emerged: night sweats, fevers, vomiting, and a marked decline in Chris's overall stamina. The onset of these symptoms raised a mental red flag. True panic had descended on our household. What followed was another series of doctor visits, where an array of blood tests were performed in an attempt to understand what exactly was going on. As we returned from what seemed like a never-ending investigation, no closer to knowing what was eating away at our son, I settled Chris onto the couch, trying to not reveal my frustration or my fear. Quietly I vowed to him that I would continue to drag him from one doctor to another until they figured out what was wrong. Questions about what was happening to my child filled my head. I wanted to scream. I wanted answers. I wanted Chris well.

I could see clearly that Chris was failing. His over six-foot frame was now weakly supporting, as of the latest weigh-in, a mere 119 pounds. Two other teens at his high school had mononucleosis, and a strange bug was also making the rounds. Blood tests came back positive for mononucleosis, but in my heart (call it a mother's intuition) I knew something worse was overtaking his body, like ten-year locusts swarming through fertile lands. I fearfully, yet boldly, asked the nurse if he could have cancer. She looked at me with a confused expression and gently but firmly reassured me that what Chris had was mononucleosis, not cancer.

Cancer had struck so many family members: two of my first cousins had been diagnosed with Hodgkin's lymphoma as teens; my mother had survived bladder and colon cancer; and my mother-in-law had miraculously survived ovarian cancer. On both sides of our family, we had experienced the loss of uncles, aunts, and cousins to cancer. My husband's first cousin was buried only miles from our home. He lost his battle to cancer at thirty-two years of age. I also had a first cousin who lost her life to cancer at age forty-two. Cancer seemed destined to cross our path. I always had a sense that I would be the one stricken with this horrible

3

disease, but I silently cried out, God, please, not my child.

Memories of my mom began to flood my mental horizon. She was friends with several moms who had lost children, and she had confided in me several times the horror of burying your offspring, when it should only occur in the reverse. I was reminded of a time when, sitting in Chris's preschool, I had listened with horror as a mom explained her young daughter's condition. The mother just wanted her daughter to experience school and wear her shiny red shoes, to be a normal four-year-old. The little girl died that year from cancer.

Chris's health continued to decline, and a desperate mother's plea led to more testing. I was the parent who panicked. Tony, on the other hand, was the "tough it up" kind of dad. The standing joke in our home was that two feet of blood squirting from a wound was required by Dad in order to warrant a Band-Aid. So while my anxiety level rose, Tony did his best to squelch the fire. But that Monday morning when I arrived home from a before-school orthodontist appointment for our daughter; Tony was no longer playing the "tough it up, put a hat on, go to bed, you'll be fine" philosophy. He had already contacted our physician and scheduled an appointment for Chris, Tony, and I that very morning.

As we entered the office, our doctor saw the helplessness in our eyes. More testing was ordered, and the next twenty-four hours were filled with an overwhelming uneasiness.

Anxiously awaiting test results, Tony answered the morning call from the doctor's office. He relayed the message that they wanted all three of us to come into their office at 10 a.m. I was rushing to get ready when the phone rang a second time. The message was, NOW—not to wait, but to get into the car and head to the doctor's office ASAP.

As we carefully backed out of the garage, Chris wondered aloud what Tony and I were fearing: why were they having us come into the office and not just telling us the test results over the phone? Tony and I concealed our fears as I pushed the CD button to track eight: "Carry Me" by Amy Grant. My friend Debbie had been urged by the Lord to give me this song and it had become a musical sanctuary over the last few days. Now the three of us listened intently to each word of the song, as it united our hearts while we faced this storm, carried in Our Savior's loving arms.

Our friend and general practitioner, Greg, escorted us into a private prayer room at the rear of his office. He looked at Chris and tenderly asked whether he had ever heard of leukemia. Chris muttered, "Yeah, it's a cancer."

Dr. Greg explained that the latest blood work now revealed that cancer, possibly leukemia, was the reason for his sickness and not mononucleosis. We were instructed to head immediately to the hospital for further testing and a definitive diagnosis—immediately was the operative word. I clumsily stammered to take control of something, anything! So while Tony helped Chris to the car, I requested copies of his latest blood work. I wanted to feel like I was doing something useful. While holding back tears, I scurried to the parking lot—and was paralyzed by what I like to call a "Snapshot from God," a memory that God would imprint on my heart. There in the parking lot stood my husband and our gaunt son, who now towered over his father, tearfully embracing. We were united; we were a family; we would survive—and I knew at that instant that God was in our midst, and that He would carry us through this storm.

*   *   *

The hospital was less than a mile from our doctor's office. In the three years we had resided in Charlottesville, I had set foot in the hospital only once: to escort someone to the volunteer services. I was now at the beginning of many long seasons of learning the ins and outs of the University of Virginia Hospital.

We entered what would soon become an all-too-familiar setting: the pediatric primary care clinic. Upon entering the clinic, we were quickly ushered into a private room. We could feel a sense of urgency; all systems were a "go." The staff had been alerted to our arrival. There was no lingering in the waiting room. No forms to complete. The hospital staff knew their roles and worked in an expedient manner, like a well-oiled machine. Despite my nervousness, I felt a sense of well-being—I felt confident that this was where we needed to be.

I carefully asked the nurse, not wanting to disturb her but needing to know, what to pray for. She did not hesitate; she did not bat an eye. She had held this position for twenty-six years and she had seen it all. She confidently whispered, "Pray for Acute Lymphoblastic Leukemia, precursor B." The veteran nurse, whom I grew to love and trust, and whose name was Pat, calmly explained that of all the illnesses Chris could have, acute lymphoblastic leukemia or "ALL," had the highest survival rate. So I stumbled, as if I were in a stupor or had spent the night revved up on caffeine, unable to sleep, searching the unfamiliar halls in hopes of finding a phone I could use to contact our church to request prayer for our son to have a specific type of cancer—a reality I was still not able to absorb. I walked in a daze back to our new station. It was surreal, as if I were dreaming. We struggled to pray, we tried to hide our fears, we sat in silence waiting for the test results. After MRIs, bone marrow tests, and scans, our first prayers were delivered— the acute lymphonlastic leukemia, precursor B diagnosis was confirmed.

The oncologist laid out the realities, with no sugarcoating. Chris, who had just celebrated his sixteenth birthday, was considered at higher risk due to his age. "His age?" I blurted. "You must be mistaken! He just turned sixteen. How could that be possible?" What was she talking about? She went on to clarify that after age eight, we stop building marrow in certain bones; hence, children over the age of eight have a decreased chance of survival. *Survival, cancer, our son*—my head was spinning and I felt faint. His bone marrow test revealed a one hundred percent tumor burden. He was no longer producing white blood cells to fight infection, red blood cells to carry oxygen and nutrients to his organs, or platelets to assist with clotting. We were being hit with a hard reality. We had to dig deep to find the coping mechanisms to take on such facts. But in spite of the grim forecast, Chris's oncologist shed light, brilliant light. Despite her petite stature, she grew in my mind's eye to warrior size. She firmly—with strong, never-blinking, never-faltering eye-to-eye contact with Chris—

assured him that in a week's time, she'd have him feeling somewhat better, and in a month or more, even better. Better. We had hope. We struggled to pray and thank God for all the knowledge that had been gathered to fight this dreaded disease. We thanked God for this hospital, this team, these nurses, and these doctors.

Much later I would read in a medical textbook a description of leukemia as mononucleosis out of control, explaining why the original blood tests had given faulty readings. Chris never had mononucleosis. He had leukemia masking as mononucleosis.

As we nervously sat at our hospital-prescribed station, or escorted Chris on a stretcher to various tests, or accompanied him into a new room for his MRI (wearing earplugs to aid in drowning out the noise of the machine), I began to feel like I was drowning. Maybe I wasn't breathing. Or maybe I had forgotten how to breathe. I kept hearing a voice whisper, in a serious but harsh tone, "Why?" Why my son? Why our family?

Almost instantaneously, my mind was flooded with images of the moms I knew who had lost a child to cancer, to a drowning accident, or to suicide; moms caring for highly autistic children; moms caring for children on life support. The reality of the day-to-day struggles they faced and their future concerns for their children's long-term care was pressing in on my brain. God plainly spoke to me and said, "Not *why*, but *why not?*" *Why should our family be freed from suffering?*

Before I knew it, evening had crept in, and we were now situated in a real hospital room. As I walked into the hallway, hoping to find some air to fill my deflated body, God gave me a clear vision of His mother holding Him in her lap, and a fresh pool of blood surrounding them. I comprehended on a whole new level that my God had died for me, that my God would not abandon me, and that my God would use even this for good. *I was not alone; we were not alone.*

I strongly believe God speaks to us often through others. As the night progressed into morning, I felt God speak to me again. This time, He spoke not through a vision, but through a person: Chris's oncologist. She had walked this road with many a family, and it showed on her face. She delivered her facts as truth coated in compassion. She warned us to treat Chris's cancer as an event in his life, not *as* his life. His life was not cancer. He *had* cancer—a cancer that could be cured. My fears were paralyzing me. I wanted to hold onto my son and never let go. But her words helped me address my fears. With my husband's help, I submitted. We placed Chris in His hands and said, "His will be done." Submission, relinquishing my imagined control, has been my greatest struggle, and continues to be a daily tug-of-war; yet it has also been my saving grace.

> *"I can be changed by what happens to me, but I refuse to be reduced by it."*

> —Dr. Maya Angelou

Chapter 2
Hospitals

Mark 9:24 I do believe; Lord help me overcome my unbelief!

Eight hours had passed but it felt like a lifetime. Tony went to meet our daughter, Darcy, at school.

Darcy is fifteen months younger than Chris, but since birth she had worked extremely hard to move into the place of eldest—a position that Chris was not willing to relinquish. She knew he was sick, but she did not know all that had transpired in a matter of hours. Concerns about how our new circumstances would affect her life—our life—were quickly starting to inhabit my psyche. After-school sports, sleepovers, dinners out to celebrate all those special moments, vacations—life as we knew it would be put on hold. A new life was to emerge: an uncharted life, one that felt like we were driving a car down a steep and curvy decline without brakes. *Halt; breathe,* I spoke into my soul.

Darcy entered the room, her face filled with sadness, when my second "Snapshot from God" appeared. It will remain as one of my sweetest memories, truly a gift from God. Darcy carefully crossed Chris's hospital room and tears sprang from my eyes as my children lovingly embraced. They tearfully held onto each other, neither wanting to let go. To have the family united as we embarked into unchartered waters brought about a sense of calm, as if the seas had receded.

We were thrown into a new world—the world of IVs, transfusions, blood counts, and chemotherapy. Chris was

9

hospitalized for nearly a month. He lay motionless in the bed, hardly able to raise his hand. Two towering poles stood on either side of his bed like sentries guarding a fortress, holding multiple bags of varying colors, dripping life-giving fluids into his veins. A twelve-gauge EKG was attached to his skeleton-like torso to monitor his heart. Nurses and residents scurried in and out checking his vitals, offering us reassuring smiles.

Our family of four quickly grew to include the entire seventh-floor staff, family, friends, and my mom (fondly referred to as "Nana" by my children). Upon learning of Chris's hospitalization, she rushed to our side and became a permanent fixture. At first, Tony and I took turns spending the night, but due to Tony's work demands and the hospital setting not being the most conducive to a good night's sleep, I gladly assumed the overnight duties. Darcy and my mother became sentries in Chris's hospital room. We joyfully ate our meals, including Thanksgiving dinner, at his bedside. Darcy diligently did her homework and Tony miraculously took business calls and worked on his computer, all within a ten-by-ten-foot hospital room. Additional family members completed our circle of love. Cards, presents, videos, and handmade posters all expressing love and concern began to adorn Chris's seventh-floor room. We thanked God for all those who generously donated blood, as our son received countless bags of platelets and red blood cells. His kidneys were failing, and talk of dyalisis was constant. He had four IV lines running into his veins, as well as, the twelve-line EKG hooked up to his chest. Over the course of our stay, it signaled two ventricular tachycardias, sounding an alarm that sent nurses and doctors storming his room. I now wished I had never watched hospital shows like *ER*! It was terrifying to have it played out in real life. Our sole resource was to continually turn to God and ask for His mercy.

We learned quickly what a fighter our son was. He knew how to persevere and he did it with humor and grace. We began to see our son through a new set of lenses.

Since Chris was a small boy, he had always expressed that he wanted to be an actor. Our response was unabashedly cynical:

"And what's your backup?" He would, without hesitation, state: "Stand-up comic." Tony and I spent many sleepless nights discussing the insurmountable evidence that these career goals were not only unrealistic, but also unreachable. We tearfully confessed to each other that we had once fretted over his future, but now we fervently prayed that he would live to have a future. God was teaching us many lessons. We began a journey of living in the moment. Often those moments were like standing on the edge of a cliff, afraid to look down, holding onto the edge of His robe.

It was in the tiny hospital kitchen, which by now I was fully acquainted with, that I met a mom who shared with me her rejoicing. Her daughter, who had undergone nine surgeries in her short eleven years of life, was able to eat without a feeding tube that day for the first time in her life. It was also in this pediatric wing that a seasoned aide lovingly washed Chris's hair while he lay helpless in his hospital bed. It was where I took my 2 a.m. strolls to the nurses' station where a young and eager resident would answer my questions, helping take the mystery out of deciphering blood work. Fond memories were built during those weeks. We received an outpouring of love and support. We were functioning under a veil of prayer. Chris responded to treatment. Our faith continued to be renewed.

One of the doctors on the oncology team advised that Chris shave his head, as he was destined to lose all his hair. The nurse and I watched as Chris struggled with this news. After the doctor left, she softly spoke to Chris and said, "Wait. I have worked in this unit for well over twenty years, and occasionally I have witnessed a youth who did not lose their hair." I'm not sure why, and maybe it was because both my children were blessed, unlike their mother, with an incredibly thick head of hair, but as it turned out, Chris was one of the exceptions. His hair did thin, but he never went bald. To conceal the thinning, he donned one of an assortment of hats.

Prior to Chris's discharge, Tony and I spent a grueling six hours being trained in how to care for our son. We had to learn what to look for; when to call the hospital; when to rush him to the ER; how to care for his PICC line; how to do sterile dressing changes; and how to administer his meds, which included heart medication, chemotherapy, and all the products necessary to deal with their sinister side effects. I became the family expert on interpreting blood work and ingesting medical lingo, but when it came to the hands-on, I failed miserably. After four feeble attempts, which consisted of repeatedly tossing packages of dressing paraphernalia in the trash while two hospital staff sadly scrutinized my disastrous failures, I reasoned with my onlookers: "Tony is a star "pupil" and isn't one capable dressing changer per family sufficient?" Thankfully, they conceded. Tony was a natural at all the hands-on and I was the scientific queen, and thus, our team was born.

Chris's treatment would last three and a half years. As I tried to absorb that new fact, I envisioned his entire high school career taken from him. I tried to recall others I had known who had undergone treatments for cancer, but I was unwilling to believe that any of their protocols had lasted three and a half years. As Chris soaked in this information, he calmly asked his doctor, "What happens if it comes back?" She looked directly at Chris and said without hesitating, "We start all over."

Chris didn't flinch; he didn't panic. He asked the hard questions and accepted the answers. I realized in that instant that our son had grown; he was becoming a man. Chris was taking charge; roles were changing. I felt so proud of the man he was becoming. I knew in that instant that God had His hand on my son. I rested in that peace. My heart again rejoiced.

"The best and most beautiful things in the world cannot be seen or even touched—they must be felt with the heart."

—Helen Keller

Chapter 3
Home

Psalm 23:2,3 He leads me beside quiet waters, he restores my soul.

It was nearly Christmas when we brought Chris home. As we veered into the driveway, Chris and I smiled as we witnessed the display of lights with which Darcy and Tony had so lovingly worked to adorn our home.

The interior of our home was also primed for holiday decorating. Boxes of ornaments were strewn about. I'm not sure if it was mere fatigue or a combination of fear and insecurity at the daunting task that lay before me, but all I wanted to do was collapse into my bed and hide. I didn't want to hang ornaments on the tree. I wanted to retreat to my bed and escape. It all seemed too hard. The comfort of the hospital staff and all their expertise was gone. We were in charge of our son, and I was terrified.

I fled to my room. Several hours later, my mother forcefully entered my room like a sergeant-at-arms. She announced that I had to get out of bed. I could not hide. I had two children and a husband who needed me downstairs. I rose obediently but reluctantly and headed downstairs to find Darcy and Tony placing ornaments on the tree, with Chris watching from the couch. Darcy searched my face for approval of her tree-decorating skills, and Chris just smiled and said, "Mom, I knew you'd be okay." I thought, *How does he know, when I feel so unsure?* And slowly, putting one foot in front of the other, we moved forward.

13

*   *   *

Tony and I launched into our new roles as caregivers. Tony, being the engineer, created a computer-generated matrix armed with coded names for all the drugs we were to administer to Chris. Totally intimidated by this format, I went into a ballistic frenzy, while my mother quietly drove to the pharmacy and purchased the largest weekly pill organizer I had ever seen, or even knew existed. First obstacle avoided.

We were navigating in such unchartered waters, with so many new challenges demanding to be faced. In my need to feel some sense of control, I set up a medication station. Next, I created a prep station in our master bath for PICC line care, which included a daily saline flush and heparin injection into both of his PICC line access points and weekly dressing changes. I made copies of the "when to call or rush Chris to ER" list, and posted it on all three floors. I began to organize our new life.

Organizing was a mechanism I had adopted as a young girl. I was known to empty out my siblings' drawers and meticulously refold all their belongings. Neat drawers and organized spaces gave me comfort. I took this quirky behavior right through to adulthood. In many areas of my life, it even brought me praise. I moved into the burning forest of cancer armed only with my organizational skills and basic medical knowledge.

My need for organization heightened later in life when I became a mom, and I used my compulsive behavior to squelch my insecurities. I rushed into taking classes in prenatal aerobics, breastfeeding, and infant CPR. Looking back, I realized that none of these classes prepared me for our first parental crisis. As parents of a newborn, we were greeted with a bumpy start—more like a jolt. When Chris was home and only three days old, I finally allowed myself to observe what my husband had been trying to show me and the entire hospital staff.

I had never actually witnessed someone seizing. I had learned in my parenting classes that infants make weird movements such as tremor and startle reflexes. But as I looked down at our newborn and watched his rhythmic jerking, I knew it was not good.

Tony called our pediatrician; I made sandwiches (fear of hospital food, I guess) and packed for our return to the hospital. We spent the next nine days in pediatric care. It was as if we were now in this vast sea, storms raging, the three of us holding onto each other and allowing God to take us to the shore safely.

The doctors determined that Chris had an immature nervous system, although they could not determine why; and after three months of antiseizure meds, he was declared fine. Somehow, Tony and I allowed those memories to fade, and we were blessed with our baby girl exactly fifteen months and six days after Chris was born. My mom said it was a good plan on God's part, because we had often vied for whose turn it was to hold our baby boy. Now we had two children to hold. But one plus one in baby reality did not equal two! As a nearly forty-year-old mom, I was overwhelmed! But through the colic and ear surgeries, God was preparing us. He was strengthening us, building a team, and together we would weather the storms. We had been in training, so it did not surprise me that Tony was so proficient at all the hands-on health care. I had witnessed his emergency tactics throughout the years. I still wondered whether he had chosen the wrong career path, and if the medical world was where his real passions and talents lay.

"Believe in yourself and all that you are. Know that there is something inside you that is greater than any obstacle."

—Christian D. Larson

Chapter 4
Blessings

Count your blessings! Boy, did we ever. First, I thanked God
that He had positioned us within miles of an excellent hospital.
Furthermore, our recent move from New Jersey had freed up our
finances and nearly eliminated a mortgage; this left us able to
take on the burden of medical expenses without undue hardship.
Back in New Jersey, we witnessed a family struggling to meet
the medical expenses incurred during their daughter's cancer
treatments. Our town rallied around them, and a fund-raising
dinner was born. I knew we were blessed in our finances.

Chris chose to attend a charter high school. The one-floor
building that housed only one hundred teens was manageable
for Chris to negotiate. The sacred teacher's lounge was not off-
limits to Chris, but rather a welcome station, with a sofa at his
disposal for needed rests. The teacher's fridge was now stocked
with ginger ale to ward off nausea and Boost to help supplement
his diet. Teachers videoed missed classes, and came after hours to
tutor him when he was unable to make it to class. They even made
hospital visits, complete with sandwiches, to the emergency room.

Darcy lovingly stroked her brother's back as he lay prostrate
on a stretcher, having just received a spinal tap. The nurse
carefully observed my daughter's actions and intuitively informed
her how much she would love a hospital program called Junior

Volunteers. Darcy jumped right in, with such determination and passion. I clearly remember her first day, as she exited the hospital and headed to the car with something that had been missing for months—her brilliant smile. Darcy clocked over 350 hours in the program, was honored with the Above and Beyond Award, and now knew with certainty what career she wanted to pursue: nursing.

We were blessed with a wonderful church family, generous neighbors, loving friends, and an extended family that walked, and sometimes carried, us through our cancer journey. We saw God's hand so graciously supply our physical and emotional needs, and we knew we were blessed.

"The best thing to hold onto in life is each other."

—Audrey Hepburn

Chapter 5
Reentry into the World

Genesis 28:15 I am with you! I will protect you wherever you go and will bring you back to this land. I will not leave you until I have done what I promised you!

The doctor's final prescription as we left the hospital with our now-sixteen-year-old ill son was for him to return to school. *Really? You want him to go back to school after a one-month hospital stay, with over three years of chemotherapy awaiting him? You want to purposely place him into a germ-infested environment like a high school?* It seemed downright wrong. But further explanation revealed that teens in particular need to know their life has not ended; it has not been suspended but does, in fact, go on. Germs would enter our home the moment any of the family members ventured out into the world. Hand washing was key! Correctly reheating food was essential—which meant no microwaves, no buffets, and no sushi. We added another rule—avoid the hacking, sneezing individuals—and to the formula, we added lots of prayer!

So, off he went. On his first day back, he lasted exactly one hour. I had a new role, chauffeuring Chris to and from school. I added Darcy into the mix so she would not feel any more abandoned than she already was. Because the teens attended different schools in different directions, we spent approximately two hours a day driving to and fro. But as a wise person pointed out early in the journey, "Look at this as a golden opportunity to spend one-on-one time with your teens." Tony and I never regretted those car trips.

Chris was now considered an outpatient. For the first eight months, that meant a weekly visit to the clinic for chemotherapy, spinal taps, blood work, and transfusions. In one day, he received four transfusions. A transfusion takes approximately four hours to administer. It doesn't take a math genius to realize that is a lot of hours. On one occasion, the clinic closed at 4 p.m., requiring Chris to be admitted as an inpatient. When Tony finished work, he relieved me and took over the hospital duty. It was 1 a.m. by the time the transfusions were completed and Chris and Tony ventured back home. I thanked God that we lived only miles from the hospital and that I had a wonderfully devoted spouse. On another week, Chris underwent nine transfusions as an outpatient. I felt we must be breaking records—no one could possibly have it this hard.

As if to further confirm my feelings of woe, Chris began the phase called delayed intensification. Just as the name implies, in this phase, the doctors wait until you are feeling just like you are ready to take on life again, and then they hit you hard and fast with the chemo. They brought out all the strong ammo, and not long into this ordeal, Chris began to experience debilitating headaches.

Vomiting had already been a huge part of our lives. Puke buckets and antinausea meds were already part of the household arsenal. But these headaches were different.

Chris was due for a trip to the clinic for blood work, but in my motherly wisdom, I felt that if Tony drew the sample, I could run (yes, run—that was how we now traversed life) the blood sample over to clinic, thus minimally disturbing Chris. While at the clinic, I explained in greater detail what Chris was experiencing. It was decided that he was probably suffering from a reaction to the spinal tap, and a caffeine drip would help alleviate the head pain. Again attempting to orchestrate life, I called Tony—and not out of laziness. Anyone familiar with the UVA Hospital could attest that their parking was far from adequate. So rather than re-park and park, Tony could drop Chris off, and I would meet him curbside with a wheelchair.

Tony, always ready to step into action, got some jeans for Chris to tug on, explained the plans, and raced (he also was operating in urgency mode) upstairs to tidy up his work and get on to his next role: the dad and caregiver. He heard Chris scream out an expletive, and then he heard a loud thump. He flew down the stairs and found Chris in the midst of a full- blown seizure. Not a rhythmic jerking of the arms, as we had witnessed when he was an infant, but a full body convulsion. He drew on all his first aid knowledge while frantically dialing 9-1-1. When learning that it would be a good fifteen minutes for the EMTs to arrive, he decided that he could do better. He dragged Chris along the hallway, out the door, and, miraculously, secured him into the front seat and sped to the ER. He kept calling out to an unresponsive son but just as they neared the ER, Chris snapped at his dad, clearly, but agitated, "I'm fine!" and then fell back into a comatose state.

Their arrival at the ER was bittersweet. I felt such an incredible rush of love for my husband and how he had acted so courageously—but I was greeted by a semiconscious son with blood dripping down his face. The blood, I would soon learn, was the result of him biting down on his tongue and cutting his lip while seizing.

Skilled hands immediately guided us into a room in the ER. We cried and uttered the only prayer our mouths could form: *Jesus.* We repeatedly called on His name as we waited and held onto each other in that ER room. It was not our first, nor would it be our last, visit to the ER. Chris was hospitalized a total of five times within the first eight months of his diagnosis. So I felt pretty safe—quite smug, actually—in the fact that we were experiencing the worst. No one could be experiencing anything that came close to our nightmare.

That seizure landed Chris in the hospital for several days. He acquired a new set of doctors—neurologists—and more medication. We thankfully made it through yet another storm. However, the chemo continued, and Chris's nausea was awful. But we learned to manage, and we had a medication schedule that was keeping the side effects under control. Then, just when we had settled into our new routine, we got blindsided.

We were all gathered around a pre-dinner episode of *Full House* when I looked over at Chris and realized that he was starting to have yet another *grand mal* seizure. My mom, daughter, husband and I all witnessed this one. Chris hit his head on the coffee table as he went down. His complete blood count (CBC) the day before showed his platelets to be at a dangerous level of 20. Platelets function to clot blood in the body, and the normal range is 150 to 450. All I could think about was hemorrhaging of the brain.

This time Tony had the means of administering a drug to lessen the seizure. When the ambulance finally arrived, I rode shotgun. Chris kept crying out for me from the back, and I felt so helpless. The ambulance drivers insisted on getting his vitals, but Chris was still in a semi-seizing state, and they were unsuccessful. After hearing my frantic pleas to just get him to the hospital, they took off, but not as I expected. I couldn't understand why they were not using the red flashing lights and sirens to whirl through the one million red lights we were encountering. My inquiries were answered with silence. Dealing with out-of-control moms must be part of emergency medical training. Needless to say, Tony, Darcy, and my mom had spent nearly ten anxious minutes awaiting our arrival at the ER.

This was when I really began to feel that God was not playing fair at all. We were experiencing far more drama than the average Joe. He had it in for us. This was just not fair. Then— *wham, God does it again!* I was strolling to the hospital cafeteria to grab some coffee and was drawn to a mom pushing an empty stroller through the corridor. I make small talk regarding her empty cargo, and she quietly explained that her young toddler was having an MRI. I can relate; Chris had had several, even a special one to rule out strokes. As we continued to walk and to talk, I learned that her son had had a seizure. Seizure—been there, done that!

But God was not going to let me feel somehow superior in my troubles. I was to learn that this young child had severe cerebral palsy and was the youngest of this single mom's three children. God was showing me that I was by far not alone in this journey of suffering, and a true lesson in humility was born. It is strange how a tragedy can set you apart and how even our pride can distort our circumstances into some heroic role.

The doctors concluded that both of Chris's seizures had been brought on by a chemotherapy called ARAC. Seizures were a very rare side effect, but since Chris had a history of seizure activity, he had a low threshold for reoccurrence. They decided to eliminate this drug from his protocol. Another storm was weathered.

"Still, like air, I rise."

—Dr. Maya Angelou

Chapter 6
Death and Dying

Psalm 103:15 As for man, his days are like grass.

Chris and Darcy, like most teens, shared a morbid interest in the concept of death. Coupling their natural teen interest with our life circumstances, death became a frequent topic of discussion.

Chris first broached the topic shortly after we returned home from his first hospital stay. Tony and I were standing over his bed as he lay prostrate. He looked up at us searchingly and asked if we thought he was going to die.

My eyes burned from the tears I held back. I began to speak, but I knew that God was now forming my words and creating the sounds necessary to evoke speech. I told him that no one knows for certain when they will die. I added that the doctors, his family, Dad, Darcy, I, and all those praying for his recovery, were praying that he would die an old man in his own bed, surrounded by friends and family who loved him. I watched his face as he took in this information and I knew that he was pleased with this vision. His life had a happy ending.

On a separate occasion, a dinnertime argument arose between Chris and Darcy. Chris was adamantly affirming the stance that due to his illness, he was the closest to death in our family. Darcy argued, with great ardor and truth, I must add, that he was no closer to death than anyone else in our household. So there! Tony and I intervened with our example of a doctor who had worked feverishly to heal a dying patient, and miraculously saved the patient's life through his skill and perseverance. The same doctor, hours later, would step out into the dark street to be struck and killed instantaneously by a speeding vehicle. We felt confident that we had just settled the whole "who's-dying-first" argument. But it would be a reemerging topic that would now bring us to tears with laughter. Predicting your own death, as we learned, is not in our job descriptions.

My father had suffered for many years prior to joining our Lord in heaven. During the last months of his life, he was receiving dialysis three times per week. He was extremely weak, and one day, he was rushed from dialysis to the hospital because the doctors were unable to get his vital signs. It was then that he decided to discontinue the therapies and to let his time on Earth run its course. He knew he was dying; in fact, doctors predicted he would die within ten days, or perhaps a maximum of two weeks, without treatments. He quietly confided to me that dying was not easy. It was not a mere snap of the fingers or a wave of a wand and *poof*, like magic, life is over. Dying is a process, and in most circumstances, a process we have no control over.

My father wanted to be brought home. We immediately brought in hospice care. My father died not as predicted, but, due to our Lord's mercy, sixteen hours after he was carried into his own bed. All in God's timing.

Tony and Chris shared a dialogue early on in his treatment. Chris was angry at the time, and rightfully so, about his perceived pending death sentence—leukemia. Tony vehemently argued that death was not immediately knocking at his door, and with that fact set in place, he challenged Chris to figure out what he wanted to do with the life he had remaining, whether it be days or decades. Chris protested that in his short life of sixteen years, he had done it all. Tony's advice: start a new list. In the course of Chris's treatment, I believe that, as a family, we all learned a valuable lesson: our lives are precious; don't waste them.

"The Family. We were a strange little band of characters trudging through life sharing diseases and toothpaste, coveting one another's desserts, hiding

shampoo, borrowing money, locking each other out of our rooms, inflicting pain and kissing to heal it in the same instant, loving, laughing, defending and trying to find the common thread that bonds us all together."

—Erma Bombeck

Chapter 7
Breathing Lessons

Philippians 4:6, 7 Do not be anxious about anything. Instead, in every situation, through prayer and petition with thanksgiving, tell your requests to God. And the peace of God that surpasses all understanding will guard your hearts and minds in Christ Jesus.

Summer had now settled upon us. Spring had been a blur. Chris had made it through the roughest part of his protocol, and mid-July had ushered in the long-awaited maintenance phase. "Maintenance"—the sound of it felt refreshing. It sounded doable. I had been maintaining things all my life: households, kids, laundry, gardens. I could do this. This glorious start of a new season coincided with my yearly health checkup. It was there in the sterile doctor's office that I realized that I had stopped breathing. Not literally—but it was as if I had been holding my breath since Chris had fallen ill. I found myself suffocating as I tried desperately to soak in the air.

My doctor explained that what I was experiencing was normal. She used words like *depression, anxiety*, and *fear*. She advised I start on a low dose of an antidepressant to help me navigate through to the holidays. She called it a temporary fix. Calmly and with great empathy, she explained that I had lost my footing; this drug would help me ride out the storm.

I left the office feeling weak, defeated. I had always been the optimistic type. As much as I tried to lean into God, a deep exhaustion had taken over my mind and body. I did not resist; after all, I was one of my son's primary caregivers, along with Tony. I needed to be strong and persevere. I needed to be like my son and fight the fight. I needed to be an example for my daughter that God had not abandoned us.

I took my pill daily through the holidays. I decorated our home; I baked cookies and cooked lavish feasts, and I poured myself into my role as mother and homemaker. As January arrived, I stopped my medication. I would be lying if I were to say that depression had not crept into my life before or since this incident, but never as profoundly and never, as yet, requiring medication. I attribute it to the prayers that have been prayed when I was unable to find the words, the buoys that were cast into the waters to rescue me, and a profound belief that God is good.

This time period served as a wake-up call. Caregivers need to take time to care for themselves. This was a new concept for me. When my children were born, I felt sisterhood with the animal kingdom. I felt the lion's wrath as anticipated danger entered the path of my cubs. Motherhood made me want to put my children first. Caring for a child who was fighting a terminal illness was a huge undertaking. I needed to be physically, mentally, and emotionally strong. In order to achieve this goal, I set out on a secondary mission: strengthen the caregiver.

Tony had always been a strong advocate of exercise. I, on the other hand, classified napping as a form of exercise. Somewhat reluctantly, I joined the gym. By the following summer, I was able to bicycle over five miles of hilly terrain to the yoga studio, take a yoga class, and bike back. I was feeling strong again. Also that summer, we hosted a young girl from France whom Darcy had befriended a year prior and had been pen pals with over that time. I added gourmet cooking to the mix. I created glorious picnics that had hints of French countryside written all over them. I was enjoying life, my family, friends, and breathing in all the blessings that we had received and continue to receive.

"Take a shower, wash off the day. Drink a glass of water. Make the room dark. Lie down and close your eyes. Notice the silence. Notice your heart still beating. Still fighting. You made it, after all. You made it another day. And you can make it one more. You're doing just fine."

—Charlotte Eriksson

Chapter 8
Maintenance

Romans 5:3, 4: Suffering produces perseverance; perseverance, character; and character, hope.

Maintenance turned out to be far from a piece of cake. It consisted of four types of chemotherapy administered orally, intravenously, and intrathecally (via the spinal column). Chris took the backbone of the therapy daily in the form of oral pills called 6MP. On Monday evenings, he would take thirteen Methotrexate pills. Nausea, as Chris said, was his number one nemesis. Thankfully, we learned how to deal with this major side effect.

Chris was commissioned to the couch. He was the king of the remote. With the television under his command, there were to be no shows featuring sad stories or hospital settings—just lots of fun stuff. *Seinfeld* and *Everybody Loves Raymond* were staples. Towels and puke buckets would be lined up next to the couch. Chris would consume antinausea meds prior to and for twenty-four hours post treatment. He swallowed the pills at two-hour intervals, which, we learned by trial and error, kept the nausea at bay.

In addition to his daily and weekly regimens, Chris visited the clinic every four weeks. During these visits, he was given a spinal tap, allowing doctors to inject Methotrexate directly into his spinal column. Chris learned to prefer the injection to oral administration via pills, as the injections proved less nauseating.

During the visits, he also had his blood counts checked; received an additional chemotherapy, Vincristine, via IV; and finished off with a respiratory treatment. Many times, he left the clinic in a wheelchair. His skin was gray and he was thoroughly wiped out. On other occasions he was strong enough to lean on me, and I would get him settled at the front entrance while I went to fetch the car. I loved those moments, the times when my teenager and I strolled united in form through the hospital halls and I would softly but totally out of tune sing the lines "Lean on me when you're not strong, I'll be your strength, and I'll help you carry on." God gave us those times, and I am so thankful.

The fourth drug in Chris's regimen was one familiar to all of us—steroids. When administered in high doses as a chemotherapy agent, they actually kill leukemia cells. Every fourth week for two and a half years, Chris would take steroids for five days. He had to consume sleep aides, stomach relaxers, and acid reducers to offset the side effects of the steroids. By day six, it was as if he were coming out of his skin. While Tony and I watched the mood changes and physical ailments associated with this drug eat at our son, we wondered why anyone would electively choose to use them.

Liver complications became a big problem during this phase. During the two-and-a-half-year span, Chris's liver enzymes were elevated on nine different occasions. Each event necessitated a halt in his treatment and increased monitoring of his blood counts. Elevated liver enzymes bring on increased nausea, as if nausea had not been an already too frequent occurrence. On the positive side, high liver counts meant Chris got a break from the chemo.

We all found our roles in this phase of life. Chris received front and center stage, which he relished. Tony managed all the medications. I was the hospital transporter. Darcy helped with his weekly setup for "Methotrexate nights." We all pitched in, helping to escort him to the bathroom and rubbing his feet— another kingly indulgence that he cherished. And somehow, amid all the dread and upset that comes with illness, the postponement of family outings and vacations, and the heaviness that sickness brings to a household, we bonded. It was not easy, and it was not instantaneous, but it was such a blessing.

> *"He said, 'You become. It takes a long time. That's why it doesn't happen often to people who break easily, or have sharp edges, or who have to be carefully kept. Generally, by the time you are Real, most of your hair has been loved off, and your eyes drop out and you get loose in the joints and very shabby. But these things don't matter at all, because once you are Real, you can't be ugly, except to people who don't understand.'"*
>
> *—The Velveteen Rabbit*

Chapter 9
Bonding and Humor

Hebrews 13:2 Don't neglect hospitality, because through it some have entertained angels without knowing it.

On our first harried visit to the hospital to diagnose Chris's illness, multiple tests were performed, including an MRI to rule out brain lesions. I accompanied Chris to the test. We were both given earplugs to help drown out the thunderous sounds. Chris had a face mask placed on his head to aid in keeping him stationary. As they placed the mask on his face, Chris did his best imitation of Hannibal Lecter!

Chris worked hard to keep humor alive. It was as if laughter were part of his protocol. He developed a bantering style with all his medical staff. He used humor and warmth to fuel his relationships. As Chris received his care, I saw a magnificent gift evolve and mature in him. I believe it is a gift from God. It still lives stong in him today, and Chris has shared it with all who have touched his life—the gift of humor.

Just a few years prior, a young teen from our area had been treated for and ultimately lost his life to cancer at UVA Hospital. In his name, a foundation was established, Jeffrey's Gifts. Jeffrey's desire was that every child battling a terminal illness would receive a gift through the foundation. When Chris was asked what he wanted, he surprised us with his request for a video camera.

Chris had not shown a prior interest in filming or

photography, so we asked why. Chris explained that he wanted to make a movie about his cancer. Wow! That seemed really cool. We were excited about his project. On our clinic visit when the camera was presented to him, Tony jumped right in to assist. Chris was set up with an IV for his infusion, sedation was administered, and he had a spinal tap. Tony asked permission to film and started rolling.

Tony and I both thought that Chris wanted to make a documentary about his treatment. But when Chris was more cognizant, he explained his desire: he wanted to produce a *comedy*. Chris did not want to show the ugly side of his illness; he wanted to bring laughter to his journey. Hence, his video production, *Live, Laugh, Love,* was conceived.

Live, Laugh, Love evolved into a medley of parodies based on Chris's cancer experiences. A spinal tap was depicted in which Chris did his best rendition of a tap dancer, including a cane and top hat act. He played a mob boss calling on his chemotherapy agents to go after those leukemia cells and ordering them to make sure those cells "slept with the fishes!" He shagged the cancer in Austin Powers's style. In a *Braveheart* scene, he passionately called on his countrymen to not let this cancer take his life—or his hair!

The project helped Chris emerge from the couch and engage in life. He would come alive as he scripted, acted, filmed, and directed his videos. Tony and Darcy played in several scenes, along with others. Darcy even wrote a rap song, and Chris was now "Chemo Chris," rapping with his backup dancers and singers. I had the part-time roles of cameraman, which challenged my technological skills; and wardrobe creater—my personal favorite.

Chris created his film during the roughest part of his treatment. He taught us how to see our life circumstances in a healthy, accepting way while further strengthening our family ties. Humor was his mantra. In fact, after Chris had suffered his seizures, we were out for a family dinner. After the check was delivered to our table, Chris asked us if he should feign a seizure and see if we could eke out a free meal. We would, from that point on, jokingly state that we should play the "cancer card." No, Chris did not fake a seizure—but the lesson in humor that he displayed played an integral role in how we walked this cancer journey and, thankfully, extends into all aspects of our life. Thank You, God, for the gift of laughter; it truly is good medicine.

"When I was five years old, my mother always told me that happiness was the key to life. When I went to school they asked me what I wanted to be when I grew up. I wrote down "happy." They told me I didn't understand the assignment, and I told them they didn't understand life."

—John Lennon

Chapter 10
Music

Psalm 149:1, 3 Praise the Lord! Sing to the Lord a new song! . . . Let them praise his name with dancing . . . sing praises to him to the accompaniment of the tambourine and harp!

Music has always been a part of our family life. No, we are not the Von Trapps. We are more "the music appreciators," with a slice of performance thrown into the mix. Both Chris and Darcy began elementary school knowing all the words to Jimmy Durante, Johnny Cash, and Patsy Cline tunes, just to name a few of our car trip selections. The children played piano, followed by sax for Chris and clarinet for Darcy—all abandoned prior to high school. Tony always tinkered with the guitar, and for my fiftieth birthday, he purchased a Celtic harp, which has sadly only gathered dust. Darcy loved her choral activities and both she and Chris participated in musical performances during their high school years. More recently, Chris had the opportunity to sing and dance as he poured himself into the role of Mrs. White, a matronly housekeeper, in the play *Clue*.

Our family's cancer journey amplified music's role in our lives. Chris would strategically choose which tunes he would bring to clinic. The Rolling Stones would rock his clinic room as the agile nurses and doctors maneuvered to the beat. The question of which musical selection Chris would bring to the hospital became a guessing game among the staff. On one occasion, we inadvertently left the music at home, and a willing nurse and I joined forces to sing numbers such as "Yellow Submarine" and "Hey Jude" while Chris received his umpteenth spinal tap. Ballads from Johnny Cash and Bob Dylan emanated from our cubicle. It was a nice change for the hospital staff, who predominately saw much younger patients.

The second Christmas after Chris's diagnosis, the four of us attended a New Year's Eve First Night Celebration. At one of the venues, a group was performing Beatles numbers. We rang in the New Year together, dancing to "Let It Be." Thank You, God for that sweet memory, and the role music plays in our lives.

"Music begins where the possibilities of language end."

—Jean Sibelius

Part II

A Case of Extreme

Mother-Son Bonding

Chapter 11
Weird Happenings

Philippians 4:6 Do not be anxious about anything. Instead in every situation . . . tell your requests to God.

Spring had ascended. I was well into my caregiver-strengthening regimen when I was stricken by stabbing abdominal pains. It was a Sunday afternoon because ailments warranting emergency room visits always seem to appear on the weekends. Both my parents had their gallbladders removed by age fifty so I felt this was a no-brainer. Tony and I headed to the now familiar ER. Abdominal X-rays were taken, and the results were: distention due to gas! I received a "cocktail" to relieve the pain and we now had a new family joke to add to our repertoire: "Mom is just full of air!"

Mid-August, while still in our caregiver get healthy mode, Tony and I began a liver-cleansing treatment. A few days into the procedure I began to experience a swelling in my throat. I quickly swallowed some allergy medication as Tony contacted the poison control center. They advised me to get to the ER if the symptoms did not subside. On the way to the hospital, things settled down, and I coerced Tony into heading back home. I just couldn't face another lame visit to the ER. I was beginning to wonder if I was a hypochondriac. We had yet another Mom story to laugh about and we abandoned the liver cleansing treatment.

One week later, the same swelling appeared, and I again took an allergy med—but this time there was no way to get out of an

ER visit. Tony was too determined. The ER was packed, and to make matters even worse, shortly into our waiting room stay, the staff ordered a lockdown. Apparently there had been a shooting and the victims were being treated at the two area hospitals. The shooting was thought to be gang related, so for safety purposes, no one was allowed to enter or exit the building.

Six grueling hours after our arrival, we were finally seen. The attending determined that I was experiencing an allergic reaction, and described my throat suffering as contact dermatitis. He prescribed allergy medication and an EpiPen for future episodes, and told me to undergo allergy testing ASAP.

Allergy testing revealed nothing. The allergist was so thorough, he even had me bring in samples from our vegetable garden to use for testing. Yet after all the pricking, every test came back negative. Well, at least this time I had something, even if the cause was still unknown, bigger than simply hot air. But I began to wonder if my body was trying to tell me something.

> "Be soft. Do not let the world make you hard. Do not let the pain make you hate. Do not let the bitterness steal your sweetness. Take pride that even though the rest of the world may disagree, you still believe it to be a beautiful place."
>
> —Kurt Vonnegut

Chapter 12
Back Pain

Psalm 27:11 Teach me how you want me to live, lead me along a level path.

We were experiencing hot, hazy, humid days as the month of August closed in on us. As the dog days of summer thankfully began to wane, Chris was just months shy of the two-year anniversary of his diagnosis. We were feeling strong. Darcy, Tony, and I leisurely took long bike rides without the fear of abandoning Chris. Although he was not up to the ten-mile treks the rest of the family frequently made, he comfortably lounged on the sofa with "his" remote easily within reach. He claimed eminent domain over this horizontal throne, while wearing the Prince of Cancer crown. We allowed him this time of self-indulgence, as the suffering he had endured was still fresh in our minds.

As September crept in, the evenings began to offer a welcome hint of autumn. What also mysteriously crept in was back pain—the ailment that hounds millions of Americans day in and day out. It started out slowly, an uncomfortable, nagging pain in the lower part of my back. *Push through it,* I told myself. *You're tough.* Don't most of us whine regularly after age fifty about our aching backs? This must just be a mere product of aging.

As September neared its end, the pain began to take a greater toll on my everyday life. I could no longer lie flat, and a sharp pain moved down my leg with each step I took. I visited my doctor and received a prescription for muscle relaxers. I began taking the medicine along with daily soaks in the gym hot tub and warm pool.

The leaves began to turn to scarlet and blazing tangerine, and I began to sleep—or at least attempt to sleep—in a chair. The pain worsened. It was the beginning of October, and our home had become the hub of activity for family and friends arriving to offer their annual support for a walk to help fund the Leukemia Lymphoma Society. Darcy and Tony had been organizers and fund-raisers for this event. This year, Chris was the honoree patient and addressed the crowd. Two years in a row, he had received coverage on our local news channel, so this was a big, not-to-be-missed kind of deal for a mother. After the prior year's walk, I had written the organizers to tell them that I loved the event, but only wished the walk itself could be longer. My request was granted: this year the walk of one mile had grown to three. Each step I took that night caused my whole body to cringe with pain. I made it through the walk, nearly in tears.

The next day, I headed to a chiropractor/physical therapist. X-rays were taken, and nothing unusual was found. I subjected myself to weeks of agonizing treatments, after which I would crawl off the table. One time I literally flew off the table, the pain was so excruciating. Somehow God carried me through the pain, and even gave me a slight respite for our next family adventure.

Through the Make-A-Wish Foundation, Chris was going to experience his wish on the weekend of October 25th, and we were all included. We traveled by train to Washington, D.C. and were housed at a lovely hotel within walking distance of all the major sites. The next day, the four of us were transported in a shiny black stretch limo to a posh hotel to have lunch with one of Chris's all-time favorite people, Robin Williams. Somehow—and I know it was through the grace of God—I made it through, and thoroughly enjoyed this special weekend in my son's life.

Make-A-Wish had informed Chris that ten minutes was all they could guarantee with a celebrity. Mr. Williams graciously, and with outstanding humor and warmth, spent over two hours at lunch with us, and had us attend his evening performance at George Washington University. The fun did not stop there. We were invited backstage for a meet and greet. When Mr. Williams entered the room of fifty VIPs, he raced toward Chris, flung his arms around him, and declared "My man, Chris!" Thank you, Mr. Williams, and thank You, God, for allowing me to see my son's face illuminate, and to be able to bask in the memory of that special moment. Both Darcy and Chris loved the limo, and the driver took extra care to make our trip special with sightseeing side trips. Tony good-naturedly toted my purse throughout D.C., in an effort to minimize my back pain. Chris and I were like twins, finding respites at every park bench—a continuation of our bonding. We headed back to Charlottesville with such a feeling of life's grandness.

Now we were looking directly at November. My restricted mobility was worsening. There was hardly a position I could find that did not elicit pain. Tony made strong cases for an emergency room visit, but due to my past ER experiences and through my Internet research, I convinced both of us that the back pain was at worst a herniated disk and an ER visit was not warranted. I conceded to follow up with an orthopedic doctor. One night, Tony actually had me in the car headed to the hospital when my unending protests finally caused him to turn the vehicle around.

However, on the evening of November 15th, a Friday night, my frustrated husband telephoned the ER and demanded to know the status: "Are you busy right now and if I bring my wife in, will you run every test imaginable?" Off we headed to the ER, for real this time. I was no longer protesting; the pain was now numbing.

At the hospital, the staff began with examinations, X-rays, and the record of my case history. I'm not sure if it was the long family legacy of cancer or Tony's persistence, but an MRI was finally performed on my lower back. Nothing was seen—except for a mysterious darkness at the very top of the scan. The medical staff decided to repeat the scan farther up my spine.

Most of what happened next is a blur. I remember lying there amazed and proudly proclaiming to Tony that I was able to lie perfectly still while being scanned. I was stunned, and convinced I was cured. He bluntly stated that my lack of pain was due to the immense amount of drugs that had been injected into my veins. Although I was still puzzled over my newfound freedom from pain, I obediently followed the doctor's orders not to move, and lay

43

perfectly still as I learned I was being hospitalized. I had an egg-size tumor compressing my spinal cord to the thickness of a ribbon. The doctors said it was a miracle I was not paralyzed. Fortunately, they continued, a wonderful spinal surgeon had recently joined the hospital staff, and would be called in to remove the tumor.

My first thought was that at least now they knew I wasn't faking it: something was really wrong this time. My pain was real. I wasn't some kind of nutcase. My second thoughts concerned my hospitilization, as my mind began racing to the mom to-do list. Chris had a clinic appointment in the morning. My mother, who was living with us at the time and experiencing some health issues, had a Tuesday appointment with a kidney specialist. I instructed Tony to call in the reserves, and my sister Anne, who lived closest—about four hours east—came to the rescue. Over the years, due to Chris's illness, she had thankfully become a regular in our household.

It was Sunday morning by the time the staff located a hospital room for me. By Sunday evening, my hospital room resembled Chris's—except now I was the patient, not the caregiver. As my old-time buddy would lovingly jest, ours was an extreme case of mother–son bonding. In fact, our diagnoses were two years and one day apart. I looked over at my husband and could not imagine how he could take on yet another burden, and this time solo—and then I remembered that we are never doing it alone. I glanced around my room, which was filled with those I loved, and silently thanked God for again carrying us through yet another storm.

The next big stumbling block came in the pre-op ward. It was like a scene from some war movie: a huge space, lined with hospital beds and staff scurrying to attend to the wounded. I had not removed my wedding band since our marriage twenty years prior, and it was just not budging. This was a big deal, because if it wasn't removed it would literally melt on my finger due to the neurological hookup needed to monitor the spinal incision. They called in the expert ring remover with her bag of "sure to remove all rings" tricks. My ring was still not budging—something about my knuckle growing over time; I thought, *"Please, no more tumors!"* Finally, the surgeons descended on my hospital stretcher with an enormous pair of clippers, the type I used to attack unwanted brambles from my garden, and with two cuts, the ring was off. Free of all metal, I was quickly anesthetized and wheeled off to remove the tumor that had landed me here in the first place.

Teaching hospitals are always a major hub of activity, full of interns, residents, and attending physicians. The whole experience began to take on a surreal atmosphere. They were tossing around diagnoses left and right, along with new findings. The first theory was multiple melanoma, when they found a second tumor farther up my spine that was actually embedded in the vertebrae, causing a fracture at the site. But further findings revealed yet more surprises. Spleen, liver, and kidney metastases were uncovered. The new suspicion was kidney cancer. Despite it being the smallest lesion, they felt it would be the most likely site of origin. I had visions of a *Monty Python* skit where they came with a hatchet in hand to collect someone's liver: as they chased the terrified victim around his home, he kept shouting that he thought they would come to collect his liver after he was deceased! Next I began to tell the doctors—yes *tell* the doctors—"Why not just go in and take out the spleen? It's not a necessary organ. While there, pop out the kidney; isn't that why we were given two? And doesn't that liver just grow back once sliced into?" It all sounded logical to me, but it seemed all the doctors could tell me was, "It's just not that simple, unfortunately." When my mom received treatment for colon cancer, it had taken one year; Chris's treatment was, in my opinion, an unprecedented three and a half years. So I innocently gazed up into the eyes of the only female oncologist I had encountered thus far, and shyly queried, "How long will my treatment last?"

The answer I received still haunts me to this day. In a cold and unsympathetic manner, she calmly but firmly stated, "The rest of your life." My jaw dropped, as my mind tried to grasp just what this statement implied. I presumed it meant I was to endure some form of cancer therapy for the remainder of my life, which either translated to a heck of a lot of chemo, or a very short life. Neither sounded appealing.

My mind raced next to the thought of my death. Over the years, Tony and I had had many long discussions about what our faith really meant to us in terms of dying. If we truly believe as Christians that this world is only temporary, then why do we as humans fight so desperately to stay alive? We had both determined that no heroic efforts were to be made to keep us alive in the face of a horrific event. I felt as if I were facing a mission to walk the talk—not to fear death, but rather to accept my situation. I lay in my hospital bed and tried to conceive of how God would use my cancer for good. I fantasized that God would perform a miracle, erase all my tumors, and give me the task of revealing to the world how the Lord had healed me. Other times I would imagine that it was through my dying that I would best serve the Lord, like my cousin, who shone with Our Lord's grace as she willingly accepted her own death at age forty-two after a near thirty-year battle with cancer. But God had a different plan, as usual; He did not need my scriptwriting abilities.

My hospital room was teeming with our church's leaders and Tony began explaining the latest findings, when I looked over and saw the sheer pain in my daughter's eyes. I called her to my side and held her close as she, along with the room full of prayer warriors, heard the full extent of my disease for the first time. It was purely by accident that we had not revealed to our children the full scope of my illness in private. Facts were coming at us at lightning speed, and it is my deepest regret that things unfolded as they did. I held Darcy tightly as she wept and cried out, "No, I don't want this to be real. Stop it, Mom, please." As I drew Darcy closer and attempted to soothe her, I knew deep within that this was our new reality, and a long, rough battle lay ahead. I heard my father's words, "Dying is not easy." I realized I was not going to simply float upward, at least not anytime soon; nor was I going to be a walking miracle. God had plans for me. I was to enter into a battle. I felt extremely ill-equipped; uncertainty, doubt, and fear were knocking at my door. I prayed for His armor and His shield and held onto the most basic of truths: God is good.

> *"Hardships often prepare ordinary people for an extraordinary destiny."*
>
> —C. S. Lewis

Chapter 13
Origins

Daniel 2:21 He gives wisdom to the wise; he imparts knowledge to those with understanding.

The hospital staff began to assemble the pieces of my medical puzzle. In conversation with my newly designated oncologist, I disclosed that I had had a fibroid tumor removed while undergoing a complete hysterectomy seven years prior. The pathology report declared the tumor as pre-cancer, with a low incidence of recurrence. Immediately, release papers were signed and a sample of the original tumor was sent for. All tissue samples, believe it or not, that have been run through pathology are preserved in a tumor bank. A vision sprang to mind of a vast, temperature-controlled warehouse, with floor-to-ceiling miniature drawers stacked in domino-like fashion, housing tumor samples. Who would have known?

Next, the pathologists worked their microscopic magic, and a match was confirmed. My cancer originated from the tumor in my uterus. Knowing the primary origin is a big deal; it determines the treatment protocol. My pre-cancerous fibroid had cancerous parts, and over a seven-year period, those nasty cells had worked their way through my bloodstream and found homes in distant organs. Malignant fibroids are very rare, comprising less than one percent of all fibroids. My cancer now had a name: uterine leiomyosarcoma, stage IV (ULMS). My sister jested that it sounded like an exotic cocktail.

I was to undergo two types of radiation beginning three weeks after my surgery, after my body had gotten a chance to rest. The radiation was to stabilize the spine and halt the cancer's penetration into the bones.

Radiation is sneaky. It creeps up on you. It doesn't hurt. You walk away feeling no side effects. And then the fatigue sets in, and you begin to drag yourself to each treatment.

The doctors made a mold of my body. During my radiation therapy sessions, I would lie in this podlike cast to minimize movement. I quickly learned to bring my favorite music and an eye mask to help transport me to a peaceful place. I would envision the pod to be Our Lord's arms wrapped around me, and I would find myself peacefully dozing off.

So, with radiation behind me, Tony and I headed to New York City to see a sarcoma specialist at Sloan-Kettering. All our research stressed the importance of being seen at a sarcoma center versus a standard oncology hospital. But Tony and I were conflicted. With our son receiving treatments in Virginia, it just wouldn't be possible for me to stay in New York City to receive care.

Two close friends from my childhood met us in the waiting room and literally held my hands as we sat patiently waiting for my name to be called. The doctors listened to our situation and thankfully gave us a protocol to start at UVA. They left us with the understanding that when UVA ran out of options, we were to come back, and they would see what they could come up with. We felt an incredible sense of relief. We had a plan, and it seemed manageable.

"I've seen better days, but I've also seen worse. I don't have everything I want, but I have all I need. I woke up with some aches and pains, but I woke up. My life may not be perfect, but I am blessed."

—Unknown

http://quotesideas.com/ive-seen-better-days-lessons-learned-in-life-quotes/

Chapter 14
My Turn on the Couch

Matthew 11:28 Come to me, all you who are weary and burdened, and I will give you rest.

Chemotherapy. I felt a battle emerging, gnawing at my core. I had watched my mother go through horrific vomiting, weakness, and two ambulance rides to the hospital before doctors decided her body could not handle any more of the toxic chemicals delivered to her by chemotherapy. That was during her second bout with cancer. The first time, she had been in her early fifties—that was bladder cancer, and required surgery and monitoring. The second time, she was in her sixties, with stage III colon cancer. To combat it, doctors had surgically removed over five feet of her large intestines, and then the grueling months of chemotherapy began. I researched the benefits, and was convinced it was killing her and destroying any quality of life that remained. Although she didn't make it through the scheduled protocol, the chemo did the trick, and she remained cancer free for over a decade.

In contemplating the battle I was to face, I also knew I had to be a model of strength for my son. Chris would half-jokingly ask me to run off to Mexico with him instead of to the clinic to receive the toxic chemicals that would hopefully cure him of his cancer. He was still receiving treatment in the form of chemo daily, and whenever he broached the topic of quitting, Tony and I fiercely upheld the treatment path as the cure, the best and only option. Chris even confronted his oncologist, who, as usual, laid it on the line: "Chris, I have been doing this for over twenty years. I can get you better. If you stop, you will be dead in a month's time." To this I added a second voice—my own—coaching my son, as though he were an all-star athlete: "Do not give up." I told him we had to do this; there was no escape. End of topic. Chemo it will be. Bring it on. I am ready. I am strong. I can do this.

The plan was to try a drug called Doxil, a derivative of a drug that I was quite familiar with, Doxorubicin—aptly called the "red devil." Its trademark was its bright red color, as it flowed from the IV into the veins. Doxil, unlike Doxorubicin, has a sheath or coating on it that resembles a liposome and allows it to get closer to its target. Besides being blood-red in appearance, it also has the nasty side effect of being toxic to the heart. So, prior to starting my first round, I had a MUGA scan—a pretty cool name for a test that would measure my heart functions for baseline information.

My mother and younger sister were flying up from Florida for the big event. Tony would be meeting them at the airport, which left my older sister, Anne, to be my sole chaperone while I received my first dose.

Chemo has a cumulative effect, so I assumed round one would not be a big ordeal. I was taken to a private room—standard procedure for the first round, just in case there are any nasty side effects. They began the infusion—and unfortunately, the events that followed nearly frightened the life out of my older sister. I felt as if large cinder blocks were being dropped on my chest from above. I could feel my body levitating off the stretcher as each imaginary block landed on my chest. Things moved quickly. A red box came out, and they began injecting me with Benadryl and prednisone. My doctor was immediately summoned to the infusion center. He decided to abort the mission and retry in a week, after heavy doses of premedications were administered to offset similar side effects.

I left feeling defeated. I had failed. Was I a weakling when it came to the pain index? It appeared so. I worked hard over the next week to build up my strength, to be the warrior I needed to be. So, armed with all the necessary meds prior to round two of Doxil, and knowing I had a host of people praying for me,

I launched ahead. This time it was just Tony and I, still in our private space to watch for any weird happenings. They lowered the infusion rate, and things seemed to be going fine. I was most definitely in a loopy mode from all the premedications, and when I needed to use the restroom, I needed Tony's assistance. In the restroom, I discovered huge raised blotches of hives covering my torso—blotches six inches in diameter. In my loosey-goosey state, I didn't think it was a big deal, but thought I should mention it to my nurse regardless. Well, that caused a bit of a ruckus, and they again brought out the red box and began their injection of antidotes to offset the allergic reaction. I wasn't a wimp after all; I was simply allergic to this drug. I felt such relief knowing that. No more Doxil—my reaction was deemed near fatal. Never again would I have to go near the "red devil" or any of its relations. I breathed a silent hooray!

After two weeks spent recovering from my first experience with chemo, doctors tried a second agent. This one was referred to as gem/tax, short for Gemcitabine/Taxotere. Round one went well: no crazy side effects, no nausea. A harpist played while I quietly and contentedly received the drugs. I was in a shared space, as this protocol had been around for a while and did not require the careful monitoring that the "red devil" did. As I stretched out in my lounge chair, I conversed with my neighbor. She had advanced breast cancer and was receiving the same protocol. She explained what to expect, and that on day thirteen, her hair had completely fallen out. She was now on round four of her protocol, and looked battered from the whole ordeal.

The chemo drugs were administered via an IV over a three-week period: two weeks on, one week to recover, and then they hit you again. Just as my lady friend predicted, on day thirteen, my hair began to fall out. I had Tony take his shears and give me a really close cut as both kids jammed into the bathroom to observe. By the next day, I looked like a bowling ball. There was not a hair to be seen. I was beginning to feel like a branded woman, sporting surgical scars and a balding head. I couldn't help but wonder what lay ahead.

As it turned out, the answer was not what I had expected: fluid toxicity. I rapidly ballooned up with nearly eighteen pounds of fluid. I could only fit into one pair of shoes, which were adorned with Velcro straps. I ran a low-grade fever every day. I had painful headaches that were only somewhat soothed by placing cold compresses over my forehead. My nails began to fall off. It was a very low period for me. I was into round four of six projected rounds of chemo when my oncologist ordered a chest X-ray and decided I needed to have my lungs drained. But it was his follow-up phone call that was truly a gift. He said he thought I should stop treatments; that I had reached the point at which the costs outweighed the benefits. I listened quietly, but was rejoicing inwardly. Yes, stop. Yes, please stop.

"Never be afraid to trust an unknown future to a known God."

—Corrie Ten Boom

Chapter 15
Tour de France

Hebrews 4:9, 10 A Sabbath rest remains for the people
of God, for the one who enters God's rest has also rested
from his works, just as God did from his own works.

For the first few years of Chris's treatment, fears of roaming too far from his doctors had put vacations on a backseat for us. We did not, however, forego having fun. We hosted a youth Christmas party one week after Chris came home from his initial hospital stay. We had grand feasts with family and friends. We celebrated birthdays, anniversaries, and life.

Maybe it was our reluctance to venture away from the nest that caused our daughter such anxiety. Darcy opted out of a high school trip to France the spring after my diagnosis. Ever since we had first read the *Madeline* storybooks to her as a child, learning French and living in France had been a dream of hers. We had hosted students from France; in fact, our town had a sister city in France and did much in the way of cultural exchange. So Darcy's decision saddened me, and made me rethink our choices.

That summer, Darcy was invited to stay in France with the family of her friend Sophie, whom she had met two years prior. They began a pen pal relationship, and the next year Sophie came to stay with us for three weeks. We fell in love with her and, from a distance, with her family. Her visit had taken us outside of our cancer world into the world of France. It was fun. It was exciting. I didn't want Darcy to miss out on this wonderful opportunity to explore a new culture, so I explained to my husband that the only way we could get her to go to France was to go with her. He agreed!

My oncologist was, to say the least, nervous about this adventure, but he sensed our determination. Four days prior to boarding the plane, during an exam, it was determined that my lungs had once more filled with fluid and needed to be drained yet again. To offset any clotting issues I might have during the flight, the doctors instructed Tony to administer heparin injections to me just prior to boarding the plane. We were apprehensive about performing the procedure in the airport, but to our surprise, no one paid any attention to it. I guess it is a more common occurrence than we suspected. To add to the drama, Chris's liver counts were elevated, resulting in a reduction in the dose of his chemo pills and a decrease in his meds.

So off we soared to France. I silently laughed at the thought of arriving in Paris, the city of glamour and intrigue, *bald*—and I mean totally bald, and *bloated*. But what the heck—I was living life. I was with my husband and children and we were on an adventure. Life felt perfect.

We planned to spend the first half of our trip touring the French countryside. For our first destination, we chose the Champagne region, due to its proximity to Paris. Our first night, we sat at a booth in a small, local bistro. The clientele appeared to be an assortment of colorful locals. Darcy, loving her new role, was our interpreter. When the server asked what we would like, she said, "Champagne, of course!" All the locals, who had been scrutinizing us since our entry, turned from their barstools and warmly raised their glasses in a toast to us. As the evening progressed, Darcy unveiled to us that our server, who was also the bistro owner, was a childhood cancer survivor. She blessed us with homemade desserts on the house, and I learned an important lesson. I had wrongly assumed that this pristine countryside, this idyllic village, this life away from mine, which seemed so perfect, was void of cancer. Instead, I learned that cancer has no physical boundaries, but we must work hard not to let it invade our souls.

Several days into our escape, Chris grew quite nauseous. Armed with my cell phone as we roamed the Champagne region, I calculated the time difference and, at the right time, contacted his clinic. I reported his situation to his nurse practitioner, and we all cheered upon hearing the news: "Stop the chemo until you return in ten days." Hooray!

I have since learned how researchers determine drug doses from my now-nursing-student daughter: they find a healthy, one-hundred-forty-pound male, in his twenties, and test the dose on him. My theory is that the members of our family do not fit this model, genetically speaking. My mom, Chris, and I are lightweights when it comes to drug sensitivity and metabolism. Hence, we always seem to need lower than the recommended doses. I have found this fact to somewhat frighten the oncology world. I believe they worry that if they can't get the chemo into you at the highest dose, your odds of survival are lessened. But I believe that our bodies can tell us a lot, and when our bodies say *Enough*, that's good enough for me!

At one point during the trip, I had to venture into a pharmacy, where the helpful staff fitted me with support hose and homeopathic medicine to help with my inflammation and foot swelling. I also spent a good ten minutes prior to getting out of bed with my legs elevated on the wall. But I was determined to let nothing undermine the joy of being united as a family, as we toured this magnificent countryside and built lasting memories.

On our arrival in Paris, we received a heartwarming welcome from Sophie's family. They had a small flat in Paris and had hoped we could come to their family home in the Alsace region, but time restrictions and distance made it impossible. They wanted Darcy to stay with them from the get-go, and they arranged for our stay at a nearby hostel. They treated us like royalty. They entranced us with their hospitality, warmth, and genuine love. They particularly wanted to know what I wanted to see most. Being an avid gardener and lover of art, both as an observer and as an amateur artist, I blurted out a longtime desire to see Monet's home and tour his gardens. They sprang into action, and plans were set in motion. Thanks to our hosts, we enjoyed a glorious picnic, prior to walking the grounds. Lots of respites were allowed, and great conversation brought our families closer together.

Our hosts also arranged for a tour of Paris by night, so we could take in the splendor of the City of Lights. The next day, while her parents went back to work, Sophie was our tour guide. We sailed the Seine River via water taxi, visiting the Parisian highlights. When it came to the Eiffel Tower, I contentedly opted out, and Tony lovingly chaperoned me as we sipped wine, soaked in the Parisian life, and watched the youngsters climb the tower. Yes, climb—they decided not to take the elevator. With Sophie's enthusiasm reigning, Chris was determined to make the ascent. I believe the experience was a profound game changer for him. He was more than back in life—he no longer wanted to be the sick guy on the couch. He was more than happy to give up his reign over the coveted couch! Amen!

Now, with Darcy comfortable in her new surroundings and us fully satisfied that we could not be leaving her in safer hands, we made the long journey home. Darcy remained in France for two additional weeks, and her bonds with Sophie's family grew stronger. She later spent a month in their Alsace home, and was treated as a family member when their eldest daughter was married. The bonds between our families continued to deepen, and we looked forward to our next reunion. I firmly believe that God put us here to form relationships, and that the nurturing of those relationships is good medicine.

"Tell me, what is it you plan to do with your one wild and precious life?"

—Mary Oliver

Chapter 16
Stable Is Good

Psalm 89:37 . . . it will remain stable, like the moon, his throne will endure like the skies.

When it comes to cancer diagnoses, I have learned that there are a myriad of differences—from stages, to treatments, to individual responses. When my mom was in her fifties, she had bladder cancer. It was an enclosed tumor with no apparent spread to lymph nodes or other organs. Surgery was required, followed by a five-year surveillance. In her sixties, she got colon cancer. It had spread to her lymph nodes. Surgery, which cut out five feet of her colon, was followed by nearly six months of chemotherapy. She would need to be checked for metastasis on a yearly basis. Her colon cancer was stage III. In both instances, after treatment, she was deemed "in remission."

Chris, on the other hand, had a blood cancer. His doctors measured the cancer by looking at his bone marrow, which revealed a 100 percent tumor burden. Chris was, thankfully, a "responder" to treatment after day twenty-eight. When they rechecked his marrow, there was no evidence of disease. Hallelujah! Let's stop, thank God, and end all this poison. But no, that was not how it worked. All this meant was that the doctors could proceed on the same trajectory. A "nonresponder" would have to try other options, such as a bone marrow transplant. So Chris was one of the fortunate responders, but I still wondered: why three and a half years of chemo? The answer was relayed in a simple manner by one of the oncology doctors: "Years ago, we treated the kids for five years. Then we backed off and began a two-year treatment plan. But statistically, we had failures, so it was decided to try a three-year protocol. Unfortunately, we began to see a high incidence of testicular cancer in the boy population; hence boys are now treated for three and a half years, and girls for three." Trial and error.

When chemotherapy is the treatment plan, it usually involves one or more drugs used in combination. Trial and error has shown the oncology world what has the highest efficacy. New drugs are always being developed, and the world of oncology is in a continual flux and pursuit of what works best. For leukemia, they have done their due diligence. Nearly 100 percent of the children in the United States diagnosed with cancer are treated across the country in children's hospitals specializing in cancer. The wonderful part about these specialized centers is that they share their data. Shared data has really affected the ability to come up with a successful protocol.

When I first viewed Chris's protocol, I was reminded of helping Chris learn long division. I remembered how he had looked up at me in bewilderment, and innocently asked, "Who came up with this?" His protocol was a huge maze that involved multiple phases and nearly a dozen different drugs, with multiple avenues depending on responses. The good news is that Chris was cancer free as of this writing, and soon to celebrate his nine-year anniversary from his initial diagnosis.

I had a stage IV solid tumor cancer, which meant it had found a home in an organ other than the primary site. It was also high-grade, which made it more difficult to treat. It was a rare cancer: each year, the United States diagnoses 1.6 million new cases of cancer, and just seven hundred of those cases are leiomyosarcoma. As of this writing, they still do not have an effective treatment. Only twenty-three percent of the tumors shrink or stabilize in response to treatment, with reoccurrence on average in eight to ten months. Resection, or surgically removing the tumor with clear margins, offers the highest five-year survival rate.

In researching my cancer, I would run across the acronym NED. It was puzzling for a while until I figured out its meaning: *no evidence of disease.* The sound of it was so appealing. It had hints of remission, even cure, written all over it. Unfortunately, in my case, NED has not happened, so I now have a new love: *stable*. Yes, "stable is good," as my oncologist reminds me. I like to think of it as my tumors "behaving." They are not finding new homes, like a gang of field mice, and they are not growing; rather, they are content just hanging out. So, stable is *good*. I have had many stable periods over the years, and I am so thankful for those times when cancer takes a backseat!

> *"I like living. I have sometimes been wildly, despairingly, acutely miserable, racked with sorrow, but through it all I still know quite certainly that just to be alive is a grand thing."*

> —Agatha Christie

Chapter 17
Mom

Isaiah 66:13 As a mother consoles a child, so I will console you.

My mom had become a regular at our home from the moment Chris was diagnosed with cancer. My children were her youngest grandchildren by ten years, due to my late entry into parenting. She had tenderly sat by Chris's bedside when he was hospitalized for seizures as an infant.

During that early hospital stay, we never left Chris alone. We coaxed him into wrapping his undersized hand around our index fingers. My mother was a substitute hand-holder whenever Tony or I could not be present. They formed a special bond during those hand-holding sessions, as we attempted to create a human lifeline while praying over the crib of our three-day-old son.

My mom and dad and our entire extended family warmly welcomed my children into the flock. New babies bring such a joy to our family, especially after a ten-year hiatus. When my children were just starting grade school, my father, after a long struggle with heart disease, was received into heaven at age seventy-two. My mother posted on her fridge: "I know where you are; I am the one who is lost." But she was a strong woman and, after much grief, she was able to recover her footing and gracefully march back into life. By the time Chris was diagnosed with leukemia, she had become, as we all joked, a nomad. She now traveled among her four children, not wishing to hurt any of us by choosing whom she would live with. She was the kind of mother whose children and their spouses all wanted her to reside among them. So my siblings and I conceded that when she was no longer able to traverse the east coast from one child's home to the next, she would simply reside wherever she landed last.

When illness fell on our home, our family became the mother monopolizer. She continued to make the rounds, but we definitely received the lion's share of her time. Her downward health spiral accelerated when I was first going through chemo. She was hospitalized several times, and thus acquired a slew of health care professionals who made regular visits to our turf. On one return from a hospital stay, as we gently escorted her into the house, she gleefully exclaimed as she eyed the sitting area, "It's my turn on the couch!" She combined humor with an elegant sense of proficiency.

In the last years of her life, her mobility issues grew as her third cancer, chronic lymphoid leukemia, ate away at her immune system. It was hard for my siblings to come to terms with her residing with their cancer-stricken sister. All suspicions of inadequacy were soon displaced when they saw how caring for my mother became an integral part of my protocol. It was as if God were keeping me alive for the sole purpose of being my mother's caregiver—but I was not by any means alone in this role. My husband, children, and siblings were also her caregivers. Whenever I had a surgery, doctor's appointment, or tests, my sister Anne, who lived closest, gladly made the trip; and whenever my siblings visited, they insisted that Tony and I have a special night out.

My mother went to meet her Maker on June 8th, 2012. We were planning our trip to NYC to settle Chris into his new abode at film school on July 5th. I was scheduled for kidney surgery on the 13th of July. On top of that, Tony's mom had suffered a stroke in May, and he was regularly driving more than five hours to help his dad out with his mother's care. All of this weighed heavily on my mother. As she neared death, she often expressed concern that she was too great a burden and that we should put her in a home. I would quip back that she was in a home—our home, her home. I believe that she strongly reasoned with God to please take her, so she would not be any further trouble.

I had become so comfortable accomodating my mother that I hadn't even realized how much she was failing. During the last months of her life, we ate all our meals downstairs with her. I helped her dress and bathe. She would often look at me in awe and proclaim that the doctors must have it all wrong—I couldn't possibly have all this cancer running through my body. We would laugh and we would cry together, and I miss her dearly. After she died, I went through a period of wondering what my purpose was now that she was gone. Why was God keeping me alive? My mother had pondered that same question and concluded that she must have been a very bad girl, because God didn't want her. But I think God knew how much we all wanted her, and He allowed her to live and see eight grandchildren and twenty great-grandchildren be born. She loved us all with unwavering commitment.

Cancer gives us time to reflect not just on our lives, but also on our passing. As time went on, I found myself no longer fighting the cancer, but submitting to God's will and praying for His mercy. Over the last few years, I attended numerous funerals, many for newly made friends who had cancer—"cancer buddies," brought together by life's circumstances. At such times, I couldn't help wonder why I was still here.

> *"Life is eternal, and love is immortal, and death is only a horizon, and a horizon is nothing save the limit of our sight."*

—Rossiter Worthington Raymond

Chapter 18
Jack the Knife

Jeremiah 29:11 "For I know what I have planned for you," says the Lord. "I have plans to prosper you, not to harm you, I have plans to give you a future filled with hope."

Fortunately, after chemotherapy I experienced one year without tumor growth. However, after that time period, problems began to proliferate. All my research on sarcoma, a solid tumor cancer, led me to one conclusion: if at all possible, cut the tumor out with clear margins. I talked with my oncologist about surgery on my liver and kidney, and asked for a consult with a liver surgeon. As we anxiously awaited the arrival of the consulting physician, in walked three individuals, all cloaked in white lab coats. In as nice a way as possible, the head of the liver department asserted that I was in no way a candidate for any type of surgery on my liver. His rationale: I had too much cancer brewing throughout my body. Sitting in the office surrounded by white coats, I no longer registered the words coming out of his mouth. My only focus was on the opening and closing of his lips. I was overcome with the sensation of numbness. Deep down, I sensed that this was not good news.

I left that visit feeling defeated once again. My one ray of hope had evaporated. But after several weeks of feeling depressed, I began to rethink my situation. With a new sense of determination, I requested copies of my entire health record. After carefully scrutinizing the data, armed with highlighters and Post-It Notes, I surmised that my cancer was only active in two places: my liver and left kidney. Therefore, I felt reasonably certain that I was indeed a candidate for surgery. Now the tricky part—convincing the doctors.

In a very self-assured manner, with data in hand, I met my oncologist, who granted me an hour-long visit to state my case. Together we scoured the records and indeed, came to the mutual conclusion that my body was not riddled with active disease. He informed me that the next step was to bring my case to the tumor board for a comprehensive evaluation. I envisioned a long wooden table encircled by a sea of white coats ruling on my fate.

It was as if the stars and planets were all in alignment. The head of the liver surgery had left on medical leave, and his replacement, an eager young surgeon fresh from the Mayo Clinic, was anxious to get his hands on my now-15.6-centimeter liver tumor, which was about the size of a cantaloupe. The removal was not a one-two-three deal, but would require a series of intricate surgical procedures.

Due to the size of the tumor and its placement, I had to undergo a preliminary procedure called portal vein embolization, which entailed entering the portal vein and cutting off the tributaries supplying blood to feeding the liver. The hope was that the remaining tumor-free, healthy liver lobe would be tricked into growing, thereby increasing the size of the liver that would remain after the resection. For the size of my tumor and the amount of necessary resection, this amounted to an eighty percent blood supply shutdown. The procedure took two doctors working in tandem for a total of four hours. After three weeks, voilá, the healthy liver had grown fifteen percent. Now I was a viable candidate for liver resection.

My next hurdle was the resection of sixty-five percent of my liver. The surgery took nine hours, and was followed by a grueling recovery process. To achieve its original volume, my liver was set to the task of regeneration. I would be forever destined to house a functioning lopsided liver, as opposed to a normal two-lobed liver.

I soon learned to appreciate the liver's role in metabolism

the hard way. In between vomiting bile and dealing with a twelve-inch incision, my poor body felt as if it had been run over by a Mack truck. But I was not deterred: my kidney surgery had been scheduled for seven weeks after my liver surgery, and I was afraid to alter the time schedule, lest they might change their minds.

After the liver ordeal, the kidney surgery was a piece of cake. The kidney surgeon lovingly nicknamed me her "poster child." I emerged with flying colors, and within weeks, I was back at the gym. These surgeries granted me an eighteen-month stretch without significant tumor growth. As I like to phrase it, "my tumors were behaving"—but not for long. My surgical respite came to a halt when my jealous right kidney demanded resection. The four-centimeter tumor was removed with relative ease, and after several weeks of recovery, I was back in the gym.

I began to have déjà-vu shooting pain up and down my spine only a few months after my second kidney surgery. Flanked with spinal spasms, I went to see my original spinal neurosurgeon. He explained in cold scientific terms that without intervention, I would be paralyzed and in a wheelchair in six months' time. So with limited options—surgery or no surgery—I fearfully chose the surgery.

But this surgery was a far greater ordeal than anything I could have ever imagined. It required the removal of two vertebrae, T-7 and T-8, and the insertion of two twelve-inch rods, fourteen screws, and an expandable cage. This particular nine-hour surgery landed me in the ICU, followed by a seven-day hospital stay. Physical and occupational therapists visited my hospital room in an attempt to determine how I would perform activities of daily living once discharged. Their assessment led to orders for a walker and confinement to one floor. Stairs were forbidden. Needless to say, I did not make it to the gym. But I was determined to live, and living required resilience. My first night home, I trudged up the stairs to my bedroom with perseverance and frequent rests. While the walker accumulated dust in my closet, I slowly regained the strength necessary to take short walks and eventually mount my bicycle.

My final surgery was a "simple" day surgery to remove

a tumor from my scalp. Although it was one of my smallest surgeries, it was the hardest for me to cope with. I was left with an approximately two-by-three-inch crater on my head, where hair would grow no more. It seems silly, but my vanity had been hit hard.

The ultimate question: if I had a do-over, would I opt for these surgeries again? The answer: yes. These surgeries granted me time. I would not have had the opportunity to write this book if I had not had my liver resection. No one can live very long with a 15.6-centimeter tumor growing in their liver. So thank You, Lord, for all the surgeons and nurses who skillfully perform their tasks, day in and day out, who give patients like me the gift of time.

"You gain strength, courage, and confidence by every experience in which you stop to look fear in the face. You are able to say to yourself, 'I have lived through this horror. I can take the next thing that comes along.' You must do the thing you think you cannot do."

—Eleanor Roosevelt

Chapter 19
Alternatives

Romans 6:4 . . . we have been buried with him through baptism into death, in order that just as Christ was raised from the dead through the glory of the Father, so we too may live a new life.

When you have cancer, well-meaning folks send you every possible diet, herb, and practice that proclaims to cure it. Being the good patient, I can honestly say I have spent endless hours researching their leads, as well as those I uncovered myself.

I flew out to an integrative cancer center in Chicago on the first year of this journey. They took twenty-one vials of blood. They checked my trace mineral levels, calcium counts, vitamin levels, and a slew of other blood components. I met with a psychologist, a nutritionist, and two oncologists. They started me on a supplement regiment and a vitamin D prescription. They were glad to hear I was scheduled for liver and kidney resections, as they concurred with my findings—the best possible course was to cut it out and hopefully get clear margins. I began to swallow nearly sixty pills throughout the day. I joked that I had the most expensive urine in the whole state of Virginia.

On one occasion, we found ourselves lost and quite confused trying to locate the liver surgeon's office. Out of nowhere, a kind woman appeared and got us to the right location. During our time together, she explained that her knowledge of the convoluted west wing building was the result from years spent with her brother.

She went on to explain that he had been told he had only months to live, but had astounded the medical team by living three years. She went on to say that he had a rare cancer, a type of sarcoma!

I took this all in with a sense of awe. Sarcomas make up one percent of all cancers. There are over thirty different types of sarcomas. As the elevator closed and our time together ended, she spewed out the words "Pau d'Arco."

Believing there are no coincidences, I investigated Pau d'Arco, a bark from a tree in South America. We ordered a shipment from Canada, and Tony lovingly brewed it in a huge canning pot and transferred the liquid into sterilized quart containers. Each batch consisted of a ten-day supply. I would ingest a quart daily. We added this to my daily pill intake for a year and a half.

In addition to my cocktail of supplements, we ate organically; processed foods, white flour, and white sugar were totally taboo. The kids coined a new nickname for me: "the food Nazi!"

As time passed, scans revealed more cancer and we switched things up, truly believing cancer gets smart and we needed to readjust our strategies. I easily adopted the new methods, except for one: organic coffee enemas! I rationalized that if the alternative strategy was creating too much stress, I should abandon it. And that is precisely what I did. More recently, I spent four months following a very strict and extremely limiting ketogenic diet. This diet was developed at Johns Hopkins for pediatric epilepsy patients. It is based on an extremely low carbohydrate intake, which forces the body to fuel itself using ketones rather than glucose. The theory behind this diet and its effect on cancer is to starve the cancer cells of glucose, their preferred fuel source. Laboratory research has shown some very promising results. Unfortunately, after a four-month trial, this diet did not starve my cancer cells. In fact, I experienced significant tumor growth.

With all that being said, I do believe there is a strong link between our diets, our environments, and our health. I think that many of the alternative treatments I tried have aided in me living four times longer than the expected period of survival. Early on in my diagnosis, I asked my oncologist what I, the patient, could do. He replied that I should eat really well, get lots of rest, and be kind to myself. In addition, I believe that advice mixed with lots of prayer are the tools necessary to walk this journey. Throughout this journey it has been my faith that really kept me going, allowing me to be thankful, to see my blessings, to feel God's grace, and to rest in Him.

"Life was not meant to be easy, but take courage: it can be delightful."

—George Bernard Shaw

Chapter 20
Staying Active

Hebrews 12:1 . . . run with endurance the race set out for us.

Staying active was another part of my regimen that proved vital to my overall health and well-being. I had begun my cancer journey biking and taking yoga classes on a regular basis. I truly believe being fit aided tremendously in my ability to bounce back quickly from surgeries, chemotherapy, and radiation. Surgeons even told me that my slimness really made their job easier. After my initial spinal surgery, followed by intense, debilitating chemotherapy, I was back at the gym. Physical therapy in warm pools and restorative yoga really got me back into life.

Consequently, after each surgery I made my way back to the gym. My last big surgery, during which I had vertebrae removed and lots of hardware implanted in my spine, did limit what I could physically do. As a result, simple walking and biking became key components of my daily routine. It was only later, as I moved into my hospice phase, that I abandoned the bicycle and shortened my walks. Nevertheless, I still try to push myself, albiet gently, to trying to find the right balance and to adjust as needed.

Breathing—simply breathing—was a key component of my lifestyle. Early on, as I delved into cancer research, I found studies on the benefits of breathing in relation to cancer. The theory was simple: Cancer cells do not thrive in a well-oxygenated body. One of my yoga instructors gave me a bumper sticker that simply reads:

"BREATHE." It served as a wonderful reminder to do just that—breathe! I even played with breathing slowly and peacefully while having my blood pressure taken. Prior to my implementation of this exercise, my anxiousness surrounding my visits to the hospital would put my pressure into the high 120's over 100. By simply breathing mindfully, I found my pressure dropped twenty points. I gained a sense of calm with this practice. When I coupled it with music and an eye pillow, I found myself drifting into a state of tranquility. I used this technique while being scanned or radiated. Often I visualized myself in my Lord's arms, protected and safe.

All of these techniques take practice. Although I do occasionally slip into a state of inertia, I try very hard not to linger there. Whenever I feel myself beginning to feel apathetic, I remind myself of the message in the movie *The Pursuit of Happyness*: happiness doesn't just fall into our laps. Instead, I believe it is a choice, and one that takes work.

"The mind is everything. What you think, you become."

—Buddha

Chapter 21
Palliative Care

2 Thessalonians 3:5, 16 Now may the Lord direct your hearts toward the love of God and the endurance of Christ. . . . Now may the Lord of peace himself give you peace at all times and in every way. The Lord be with you all.

As I lay in my hospital bed alone, in a room to myself, I had lots of time to contemplate my situation. I realized somewhere deep inside of me that this would be my last major surgery. Having vertebrae removed and their spaces filled with hardware, I knew I was not going to make it back to the gym. My body as I knew it was no longer the same. So when the nurse came to check on my vital signs, I asked, with a sense of determination if I could meet with someone from the hospice team.

Later that day, I heard someone lingering outside my hospital door. Finally, in an unsure manner, he asked me if I was Carol Alimenti. I answered that I was indeed Carol Alimenti. He explained that he had just read my chart and found it unbelievable that the woman he was now looking at was the same woman whose chart he had read. This was not the first time I had received this kind of response. But now I wanted to scream, "You don't know what they have done inside of me." I had fought so hard to have these surgeries, and now I no longer wanted them. After regaining his composure, the doctor explained that I was probably not ready for hospice, but palliative care would be a great option. This was a new word in my vocabulary: palliative. He went on to explain that palliative care manages symptoms, such as pain, constipation, nausea, shortness of breath, and so on.

Once I was discharged and had a period to recover, I asked my oncologist about being referred to palliative care. On my first visit, I saw a nurse practitioner and a doctor. When they suggested pain medication, I had reservations. I had lived with pain for a long time, and I was afraid of becoming addicted to medications. The doctors continually reassured me that I would not and that by managing my pain, I would have a better quality of life. Eventually, I did realize that managing my pain did really make for a better life. I was able to ride my bicycle, paint, garden, and hike, all during the course of the year that I received palliative care.

Toward the end of each visit, a nurse would have me work on a questionnaire. I loved that the last question I answered each time I visited my palliative team was, "What role does your faith play in your life?" My response was always the same: a big-time role! It is the main part of my protocol, it is the meat and potatoes.

"Hope is the thing with feathers
That perches in the soul
And sings the tune without the words
And never stops - at all

And sweetest - in the Gale - is heard
And sore must be the storm
That could abash the little Bird
That kept so many warm

I've heard it in the chillest land
And on the strangest Sea
Yet - never - in Extremity,
It asked a crumb - of me."

—Emily Dickinson

Chapter 22
An Endpoint

John 14:1, 2 Do not let your hearts be distressed. You believe in God; believe also in me. There are many dwelling places in my Father's house. Otherwise, I would have told you, because I am going away to make ready a place for you.

When you have a terminal disease, you often ponder your endpoint. But I always thought that I would have more time, and my endpoint seemed to stretch out so that it was a blur, not a reality. After all, I just celebrated the sixty-months-since-diagnosis landmark, well exceeding the fifteen-month average. Time—the ticking clock. I wanted the time needed to finish this book; time to paint enough paintings to have an art exhibit; the time to illustrate the children's books I had written many years ago; time to complete the baby afghans for the little ones arriving in my extended family in only a matter of months. I was even selfishly pretending one of the expected babies was my grandchild. I made videos of myself reading my own children's favorite books to share with my future grandchildren who I would not be there to hold and love. Surely I would be granted the time, a mere six months, to be present for the college graduation celebrations I was planning for my daughter.

And then the life interruption came. My palliative doctor recommended I move into hospice care. I panicked. I didn't feel ready. I had so many things unaccomplished, so many things yet to do. I hadn't made my cremation plans—the form had been sitting on my desk for the last three years. There were songs to be chosen and party plans to be made. I had vowed not to leave my husband with all the details surrounding my death. After all, I was the family planner, the detail person. I had, I thought, been on top of this dying-planning part of my life. I had attended end-of-life seminars. I had read the books. I joked that I was the most prepared dying person out there. Loved ones retorted that I would be preparing for the last event in my life for years and years to come. So my stunned expression and response to my doctor at the mention of hospice was, "But I plan to be here for my daughter's graduation." Had she somehow missed the memo?

Her response hit me like a brick wall. She took my hand and calmly advised I take that pressure off. My daughter, the stellar student, was in no way at risk of not graduating, and if my health continued on its current trajectory, we should celebrate early.

Spontaneity! It was a novel approach for the ultimate planner, a new awakening: live in the moment. First reality check: I will not get to check off all of my to-do items. Second: it's okay. Life lesson: everyone's life is incomplete. Prioritizing is what matters. What matters are my relationships: Lord, I pray for them to be healthy, healed, and happy! I pray for the grace to walk these final steps without fear. I give thanks for the gift of time that was given to me—the time to realize in my heart what truly matters.

"You matter because you are. You matter until the last moment of your life, and we will do all we can not only to help you die peacefully but also to live until you die."

—Final Gifts

Epilogue by the Caregivers

Chris

Life, oh, life, how no one had ever said it would be easy, or make anyone queasy. But in the short midst of life, there's always a blooming flower and the ray of sunshine across a baby-blue sky. Even in the depths of gloom, where the darkened gray clouded sky hovers over us, the beauty of life perseveres. Even in the shrewd darkness, a spark of beaming light shall always shine on. One must not wallow in the darkness, but grasp the light with weary hands. This is the philosophy that my mother, Carol, always tried to follow, especially when it came to trying to find and grasp tightly onto hope. Most of all, she tried to live on the bright side of life, even when the dark clouds hover and make us queasy.

My mother, with hope, the gleaming light, and her faith in God and the universe by her side like a shadow, has helped not only her live life to the best, but helped me, my dad, and my sister live our best lives as well. My mom has never given up, but has been right by my side in what seemed to be the darkest hours. Throughout my childhood, she was there for me and had never left, even on the day she passed away. At the beginning of my life, she never gave up hope, especially with my early health issues, the harsh years of middle school in New Jersey, and through the turmoil of cancer. She fought for not only me, but for my family and others, friends and relatives. She sat by my side with a caring arm around my shoulder until the day she passed. When the days of her passing came near, the cancer too hard to bear and her mind weakening, we sat beside her with caring arms around her shoulders. The tables had turned—but, still, she never gave up on me, as long as she had hope, faith, and the light of life still gleaming in her eyes.

What my mother has done for me makes my heart race like the roll of a thunderstorm. As far back as I can recall, she was right by my side. I have a recurring memory of us walking down the hospital hallways and singing "Lean On Me," by Bill Weathers, as chemo raced through my veins. She never stopped finding hope, despite the earaches I had at an early age and my seizures when I was a toddler. She tried her best to make me feel better, and fought with doctors to better my health. She never ceased fighting, even when all hell broke loose.

Later in my life, when I was in middle school in New Jersey, the teachers bewildered me, put me into a special ed program, and kept an evil glaring eye on me for not learning the same way as the others. She fought the hard fight for me and dared not give up or shrivel into a ball, but persisted in trying to make my life better. Carol, my mother, fought in court against the school board, homeschooled me so I wouldn't fall behind, and called me in sick so I could learn the information. She did all of this so I would not be pushed down by teachers and the school itself. No matter what situation arose, she stood by my side until the day she died, and I stood by her side as well.

Another memory I recall took place on a warm, sunny fall day in Charlottesville, Virginia. We drove in a silver Audi, with music playing in the background to calm our nerves on yet another of our visits to the local doctor's office to meet with our primary care physician, Greg Gelburd. On one of these drives, despite my body slowly weakening and my soul beginning to break, yet, we jokingly bickered back and forth on which song was played on the day of my diagnosis. Our disagreement centered on whether it was Mark Harris' "Find Your Wings" (my thought), or Amy Grant's "Carry You" (my mother's thought). We bickered like hens. This went on for years, but nevertheless, we enjoyed it. They were songs we shared, songs that brought meaning and hope to our lives.

Hope pushed us forward, and on November 21st of 2006, at the age of about 16, I was diagnosed with leukemia, a blood cancer. For four years, our family and my persevering loving mother with a heart of gold sat by my side. She tried her best to keep me happy during those years and to help me see the gleaming light, even if darkness hung over us. We shared laughs, made short films, and went on vacations; music always blared, and we cried our hearts out in the depths of our pain. In whatever way we suffered, we persevered in finding hope, even as we experienced great losses over the years. First I was sick, and just when I went into remission, my mother, now with severe back pain, became sick and was diagnosed with an incurable cancer, leiomyosarcoma. In spite of the disease, she persevered for seven harsh years, living life to the fullest. Whether painting, gardening, or taking vacations, she desired to grasp the light of life. Carol sat beside her mother's deathbed with cancer roaming throughout her body; she still dared not to give up yet. But soon the tables turned. Now we sat beside her with loving hands and arms guarding her, trying to keep that gleaming light in our hearts even in the darkest of hours.

No matter what situation occurred in life, our one answer was hope. Hope is the best alternative we have as a human race. Through hope, we can live life to the fullest, hope to find peace, hope to find happiness, hope we can grasp that gleaming light. Hope. Although no one ever said life would be easy or make one queasy, even a bland meal can become a thing of beauty when cooked with a dash of spices and a little love and care. That's what my mother did—she searched for the light at the end of the darkened tunnel. In the midst of a storm, when the grim clouds of gray surrounded us, as a family, we persevered and dared not give up. We searched for light, and most of all, we searched for hope.

Darcy

As I tiptoe into her bedroom, my eyes immediately narrow in on her chest. Once I see the rise and fall of her abdomen and the flare of her nostrils with each breath, I am relieved. The humming of the oxygen machine has become a familiar background noise and a blaring reminder of her illness. She lies propped on three to four pillows. Her hair is cut short, with patches where the tumors have overgrown her thin strands of silver hair. Her eyes are sunken and constantly have bags under them. The oxygen tubing fits snugly around her ears and under her chin. Her hands are held together at the center of her chest, like a praying angel's. I am relieved to see that she is still breathing—still here with me on Earth. All is good; all is it should be.

My mother has been sick for six years and eight months. She has been in hospice now for eighteen months. She has outlived every statistic on metastasized leiomyosarcoma and continues to amaze me. The wear and tear of cancer on her poor body is evident. Her once jovial, energized body has been replaced with a feeble, scarred, exhausted, aged replica. The woman who used to walk and bike for hours now calls on every bit of energy left in her body to move from her bed to the hospital bed in the family room or to the bathroom. She is fading, and there is nothing I can do to stop this dying process. I have tried bargaining with God: *Take me, instead. Leave my beautiful, hospitable, courageous mom alone.* I have tried denial: *Wow, Mom, today you were up for five whole hours. It appears that you have turned a corner.* I have tried humor: *What if I could just shrink you to the size of a pencil, and then I could carry you around with me everywhere I go and we could experience the world together?* But my humble attempts to halt the dying process are simply that—humble attempts. There is nothing I can do to stop this cancer from stealing my mother. And one day when I tiptoe in to check on her, her chest will no longer rise and her nostrils will no longer flare.

Call me Pollyanna, call me Miss Optimist, but I refuse to let that thought take center stage in my mind. Instead I choose to spend all my free time with my mother, my father, and my brother. Between my four blocks of twelve-hour nursing shifts in Baltimore, I am a permanent fixture in my parents' house. My father and I take turns sleeping with my mom, in case she needs help to the bathroom or pain medication during the night. While my mom sleeps during the day, my dad and I plan meals, clean the house, and walk. Walking has become our free form of therapy.

On these long walks, my dad and I discuss our fears of losing our prized Carol. We express anger at the unfairness of her suffering, and we cry when the pain becomes unbearable. These walks keep me sane. In the evening, when Chris comes home from work, he serenades us with his music. As the summer night comes to an end, a sweet melody escapes from my brother's guitar, and I lie next to my mother, for a moment life feels as it should. My mother would call an evening like this a "Snapshot from God," a fleeting moment that I will forever hold near and dear to my heart as a reminder that despite all the pain, suffering, grief, loss, and tears in this world, there is something bigger, better, more beautiful, and lasting to come. As we get closer to my mother's passing, this hope and these "Snapshots from God" give me the strength to get through the days. This cancer journey has been anything but easy. It has required that we as a family unite and find strength in our Lord during even the darkest moments. This cancer journey is not so much a cancer journey as it is Our Journey.

Tony

Many years, many memories, and many emotions surround "the couch." I confided in Darcy the other day that I periodically sneak upstairs to lie on and find comfort on "the couch."

A few years after our cancer journey, we moved from our two-story home with a master bedroom on the second floor into a townhome with a master bedroom on the main floor, in anticipation or expectation of Carol's reduced mobility. We conducted a major downsize, involving garage sales, newspaper advertisements, and donations; but through it all, I was reluctant to relinquish "the couch." We moved it to an upstairs room in our townhome.

It is to this place where "the couch" resides that I retreat. It is there that I sink into the embracing arms of the leather couch that held and comforted Chris, Carol, and Nana during their illnesses. It was on this couch that all of us, as a family, would sit together and hold each other. It is in the cool embrace of this couch that now I recall so many memories and experiences including not only happy times of laughter and movie watching, but also musings on the typical caregiving activities. I recall the multitude of anxious feelings I experienced over the years seeing loved ones in pain. I'd feel my heart race when I was driving and saw an ambulance or fire truck fly by me in the direction of our home. As their sirens screamed, I worried that they were going to our home. How many times in the past nine years did I feel as if my heart would jump into my throat, my fight-or-flight responses would kick in, and I'd almost go into a panic? These were years of symptom watching and hand-wringing with the doctors', hospital's, and poison control center's emergency numbers close by. I had no control of the events. I couldn't fix this. I had to rely on the doctors and nurses for their technical expertise, and on my friends and family for their sustaining prayers, thoughts, and words of comfort. I was always in a state of worry, confusion, and tentative readiness, watchful for the next emergency. When would the next allergic reaction or toxic response to some "curative" drug happen? When would I see the next fall as a result of weakness from radiated hips or surgery? *How, as a caregiver, do I comfort those I love who are experiencing unimaginable pain, sickness, and their own fears of survival?*

It would take years for this reaction to lessen in me, and for me to realize that "it will be okay, it will all work out." It took a lot of prayer on my part—and, thankfully, prayer from my friends—in order for me to find some peace. We as a family drew close. We wept together, brainstormed for solutions to patch up a seemingly destroyed life. We'd find ways to enjoy life and make good times and memories in between the moments of crisis. We laughed, prayed, cried, and made as many plans (bucket lists) as we could.

All these memories fly by my mind's eye as I rest on the couch. Given the hand we were dealt, I'm very proud of my family, and so grateful for the time I was able to spend with Carol. We have grown closer through all these trials, and our love for one another deepened. All these feelings appear to be instantaneously accessible when I lie on the couch. Thank you, Carol, and thank you for a great story and the beautiful life you introduced to me.

As I settle into the couch, these years of tears, cries, and laughter flash through my mind like a movie. I sense solace creeping over me as the ever-real reflections and fond remembrances scroll by. I sense the love and bonding of a family pulling together during the tempests of life. Many times, after a brief half hour of introspection, the couch drains the tension, anguish, and tears like a consoling parent and reminds me that it was love that overcame, even in loss. I will never get rid of "the couch," as it is such a blessing—one that held and comforted the physically sick and that now continues to offer comfort and emotional healing for those who need a little "oasis" where they can find respite from the trials of life. Even those who don't know our history are comforted, find solace, and comment on the peace they sense in spending a few moments on "the couch." I sure do.

Part III
CaringBridge Journals

CaringBridge Journals

CaringBridge.org's Mission: To amplify the love, hope and compassion in the world, making each health journey easier.

https://www.caringbridge.org/visit/chrisalimenti/

The CaringBridge website is a system we used to keep friends and family informed of our family's medical issues. It provided an easy way for us to let folks know what was going on, and to communicate our needs. It also helped us in a cathartic way, as we recorded events and news both good and bad. It started as a journal for updates on Chris; then, when their health declined, we also began adding the latest on Nana and Carol.

December 3, 2006

This CaringBridge site was created just recently. Please visit again soon for a journal update.

December 4, 2006

Monday, December 4th, Chris started the day at clinic having blood work. Praises abound, all his stats improved. For all those medical folks his ANC was 1500!!!! Chris spent a little over an hour back at school. He received a great reception from his teachers and classmates. Tomorrow it's off to school for an hour or two. Wednesday it's back to clinic for a round of chemo. Thanks again for the prayers. God is so good!!!

December 9, 2006

Saturday, December 9th, Chris did great with his chemo this week, minimal side effects. Another praise, the kidney team felt there was no permanent damage and in 2 weeks they would take him off the bi-carb and high blood pressure medicine. So far his platelet count has remained well above 30 and he has not needed to receive extra. On Friday he actually put in close to three hours at school. God is good! Next week, Wednesday the 13th, another round of chemo. Thank you again for your prayers, love, and support.

December 13, 2006

Thank you all for the wonderful notes in Chris's guestbook. We feel so blessed to be living 2.5 miles from UVA Hospital. We have met other families who have to travel two and one-half hours to get to clinic. We are also so thankful for the wonderful staff at the hospital. Chris had chemo today and again things went smoothly and he was able to go spend 3 hours at school. A real positive— Chris actually looks forward to school! His platelets were up to 43 today and his ANC was 1302. These are good numbers for someone undergoing aggressive chemo. Our next big day is Thursday, the 21st. Chris will have a bone marrow test, a spinal tap, and receive chemo into his spinal fluid. Our prayers are that he will remain a rapid responder, (blasts under five percent), an ANC of greater than 750, and no "Philadelphia" chromosomes. Again, thank you for all your prayers, love, and support.

December 22, 2006

Chris did great on Thursday. Although we do not have an official report, they feel confident he is still a "rapid responder." His chromosomes showed NO abnormalities. And his ANC is now well into the normal range, 3540!! Chris will not start his next phase of treatment until the 28th, therefore, on his sister's fifteenth birthday we will not be visiting the hospital! Alleluia!! Because we live so close to UVA, they are going to closely monitor Chris on the 28th rather than hospitalize him!! God is sooooo good. The next phase is quite intense. Twenty-two days followed by a week off and then it repeats. Prayers needed during this phase are: No bottoming out of blood counts, No flu-like symptoms, No fevers or infections, No irritation to the bladder wall, For Chris's bone marrow to work hard to build new red blood cells, which the chemo has destroyed. This phase will involve six chemo drugs administered in various ways from IVs, pushes, oral, and four spinal taps. You can view Chris and our youth group leaders' production of *A Christmas Carol* at www.eunseen.com. Wishing you all a Merry Christmas and thank you all for your love, prayers, and support.

The Alimentis

January 2, 2007

Happy New Year. We received great news on the 25th Chris's bone marrow & spinal fluid showed no leukemia!!! And today the kidney doctor began weaning Chris off of the blood pressure medicine. These are answers to prayers, so thank you all so much for faithfully praying for Chris and our whole family. However, due to the regenerative properties of leukemia cells, the chemo must continue. On the 28th, Chris started a rough phase of treatment called Consolidation. This phase really brings his blood counts down. Today he received two pints of blood. Tomorrow he will receive two more pints and have a spinal tap. So we are experiencing some long days at clinic. We continue to ask for prayer that Chris will not get an infection, fever, and/or need to be hospitalized during this phase. We are blessed and thankful for all the continued prayers and support. God Bless you all.

Love,
Carol, Tony, Chris, and Darcy

January 17, 2007

Chris is almost into the halfway mark of this phase of treatment. As this is a tough phase from a chemical dosage perspective, his red/white and platelet counts drop and he runs the risk of infections, fever, and the associated issues with those things. Last night (1/16) Chris started running a fever around 5:30 (he had been very nauseous for the past week and the medicines to address that haven't been as effective). As his temperature started to climb to the levels the doctors told us to watch for, we took him in to the ER per the instructions we were given. They started him on antibiotics right away as they try to determine the cause as either viral or bacterial. He had a reaction to the antibiotic, which they contained. Eventually he was given a room @ ~ late. M. Carol stayed overnight and I'll be going in this morning. As I [Tony] don't (as of this time) have any updates beyond this, I don't know the latest status. I didn't get a phone call in the night so I assume things are going as planned. Please continue to keep Chris and the family in your prayers. You all have been so supportive and we thank you for that help. It is only through your prayers of intercession and the grace of God that we are sustained through this trial.

Love and God Bless you, too!
Carol, Tony, Chris, and Darcy

January 20, 2007

Yesterday Chris was discharged from the hospital!!! Thank you all for your prayers. It turned out to be a virus, the stomach one that has been going around. He will be at clinic on Monday for a spinal tap and some chemo and that will end his first half of Consolidation. They will start back up with an encore in about a week's time, as soon as his counts come back up. But there are always praises. We are so thankful to God that it was not a bacterial infection, that his platelets are coming up on their own, that there were NO kidney complications, and that we are home for the weekend. Continued prayers that Chris's blood counts will continue to rise. Specifically, an ANC above 750 and a platelet level above 75.

Love and blessings to all.
Carol, Tony, Chris, and Darcy

January 27, 2007

On Friday morning Chris had a seizure. Thankfully, the MRI and CAT scan are both normal. And all his blood counts are good, in fact his ANC is 1200 and his platelets are 180!! In addition, his electrolytes are all good. He had been feeling nauseous, tired, and had headaches since his last spinal tap on Monday. His EEG shows a seizure disorder. They started him on seizure meds and he had a good night. He was discharged today. They think the chemotherapy and spinal taps, coupled with his low threshold for seizures, caused the incident. They plan to proceed with his therapy as planned on Monday. They will administer the seizure meds during his treatment and monitor the situation closely. He is weak and very tired but we are so glad to have him home and we will be watching for effects from this seizure medication. We also are praying for nausea, headaches, and tiredness to subside. He has been through quite an emotional and physical ordeal, and we are praying that he stands strong and continues to fight his Goliaths. Thank you for joining us in prayer and helping us fight this battle. With God in command we make an awesome army!

God Bless.
Carol, Tony, Chris, and Darcy

February 3, 2007

Chris had a week of tiredness as he got through some rough phases of this treatment. Yesterday he received two pints of blood and the positive effects were apparent by evening. His appetite was good and so were his spirits. Today we are going to see a matinee, *The Pursuit of Happyness*!! God is good. Monday he repeats the chemo and we know that the prayers you pray for him are what help him fight and persevere. We are so thankful. We see God's blessings each and every day through your love and prayers.

May God bless you.
Carol, Tony, Chris, and Darcy

February 6, 2007

We had clinic yesterday and Chris started another week of some rough chemo. Thank the Lord, his blood counts were all up, no transfusions needed. So it is a great way to begin this week's treatments. We also met with neurology yesterday and all the test results were good. They will continue with a low dose of meds for a year or two. This was a great praise. So thank you for all your prayers. God is so good. Chris is really wiped but he is hoping to make it to school this afternoon. We are praying that he begins, even if it is only an hour at a time, to get back into the classroom. His classmates and teachers have been so supportive and right now he needs to know his life is far from over. Please pray that he will persevere. We love you all. May you all feel God's blessings this week and rest in His love.

Carol, Tony, Chris, and Darcy

February 13, 2007

This past weekend Chris was feeling great. He received two pints of blood on Friday and we are so thankful to all the donors. Yesterday Chris had his clinic visit. His ANC, which is his infection fighting count, was an outstanding 1380 and except for a low platelet count all his other counts were up. He received two bags of platelets and made it to school by 3. He was able to partake in his school's after school African drumming program and see his friends. Chris has been in good spirits and has been really able to keep up with his school assignments. Consolidation phase is nearing an end. Chris will receive one more dose of chemo on Monday the 19th. If his counts remain up, he will begin Capizzi on the 26th, which is a fifty-seven-day, more easily tolerated phase. So we have lots to be thankful for and we see God's blessings continually. We do have a prayer request for discernment for the doctors. They are trying to determine based on MRIs whether a round of radiation should be administered. We thank you all for your continued prayers and may you all be blessed and may you all see God's blessings in your own lives. And may you know that you are all incredible blessings in our lives. God Bless!!!

Love,
Carol, Tony, Chris, and Darcy

February 15, 2007

God is so GOOOOD!!! The doctors around the nation who consulted with Chris's oncologist regarding the MRIs have unanimously concluded that radiation is not necessary. Thank you all for those prayers. God is listening!!! Today Chris got two more bags of platelets. For unknown reasons Chris seems to be a low platelet producer. Tony will drop off blood tomorrow as they suspect he will need two pints before he goes into the weekend. He is at school as I write and his spirits are great. May your day be blessed.

Love to all.
Carol, Tony, Chris, and Darcy

February 19, 2007

Chris had clinic today. We were there for a mere two hours. This is a record breaker. Last week we were at clinic four times. He [Chris] received five bags of platelets and two pints of blood, had two different chemos administered, and had an allergic reaction to one. Consequently, on several days we closed clinic. But God was so wonderfully orchestrating even the snow days so that Chris remains nearly current in all his subjects. He even got to spend some time at school seeing friends. He had several visitors. And best of all he needed NADA transfusions today. Thank You, God. For our God is a GREEEAT GOD!!! Chris is officially done with Consolidation. Hooray!!! We drop off blood on Thursday to check counts and he starts Capizzi (Chris likes the Italian sound of it and we have been told it is a much easier phase). So again thank you for your faithfulness and to God we give the glory. Our prayers this week are for Chris's blood counts to build. His ANC is improving. Thank You, Lord, in advance for all the prayers You have answered and will answer. I thank You for this army of prayer warriors carrying us through this journey. Thank You, Lord, for Chris's spirits, which have been so alive! I pray that Tony, Darcy, Chris, and I can cherish this journey and not "waste" this experience. Thank You, God, for Your grace, Your mercy, and Your people. I pray, dear Lord, that Your grace and Your mercy flow like a river into all Your people's lives. And we shout blessed be the name of the Lord.

Love,
Carol, Tony, Chris, and Darcy

March 1, 2007

Chris's next phase of treatment has been delayed. His counts are coming up but slowly. His ANC was 280 yesterday and needs to be above 750 to begin Capizzi. Praises that Chris has **NOT** needed any transfusions this week and his platelet count has risen to an astounding 139 from 62. We feel God is allowing Chris to have a breather so that his body can slowly repair and get ready for the next battle. Chris has been going to school every day this week for at least a few hours. He has made it to the gym 3 times this week. Most importantly, Chris's spirits have been great. Thank You, Lord, for being our Healer, Savior, and Comforter. And thank You for Your army of prayer warriors. God is listening. May each of you feel His blessings in your own lives this week.

Love,
Carol, Tony, Chris, and Darcy

March 5, 2007

Today Chris started Capizzi. His ANC was 1030. So thank You, God, and thanks to all you faithful prayer warriors. Today consisted of three chemos, two were injections and one was given via the spinal tap. He has been very nauseous but with each hour he seems to be feeling better. He has no additional treatment for ten days!!! May you all have a blessed day and thank you again for your prayers. God is listening.

Love,
Carol, Tony, Chris, and Darcy

March 9, 2007

Chris has had a difficult week so far. This was a bit of a bummer as we thought we were entering an easy stage. The spinal tap mixed with the Methotrexate seems to really do him in. He was unable to lift his head for days, very nauseous and vomiting lots. Wednesday we went to clinic and he received some IV fluids. They checked his chemistry and all looked good. So this week he didn't make it to school at all. But he was able to get some work done thanks to the Murray Staff and technology!! He started today with a nasty nosebleed. Tony drew blood and raced it over to the hospital. But thank You, Lord, his counts were all good. And as the warm weather is predicted to usher in this weekend, we are very hopeful that Chris will move out of this phase. As I write he is bouncing between watching *Casualties of War* and *Full House*, has kept down a large bowl of elbow noodles and is smiling!!! Another battle won! And no more chemo till Thursday and no spinal taps for a few weeks. Thank You, Lord. Now I'll go and bug him to get off the couch and take a walk around the block with me!

Love and blessings to all.
Carol, Tony, Chris, and Darcy

March 17, 2007

Happy Saint Paddy's day!!! Chris's treatment on Thursday did bring on nausea and tiredness, but thank You, Lord, it has quickly passed. Today we enjoyed a full day, a Staunton matinee at the Blackfriars Playhouse and O'Neill's in C'ville for some Irish fare. Chris was reluctant to go and was worn out by the end of the day, but admitted he had fun and was glad for the outing. No chemo till the 26th, so he will have lots of time to get strong. Thanks for all your prayers. We love you all and pray that you feel God's hand upon you and know you are His beloved.

Love,
Carol, Tony, Chris, and Darcy

March 26, 2007

Chris had a great weekend. He had lots of energy mixed with some beautiful weather. Today we spent the morning at clinic. They thought based on his counts from last Thursday that he would need a few pints of blood. But thank You, Lord, Chris's counts were great! He received two chemos and there was a noticeable change in his complexion and energy level but he made it into school for a few hours, has been able to eat meals and even had some friends over tonight. We are very hopeful after today that this round of chemo will be fairly tolerable. Due to the holiday schedule I asked if we could delay the next treatment to the 9th instead of the 5th. They were okay with that so he not only has a long stretch to recoup but can enjoy his cousins, aunts, and uncles who will be with us for the holiday. We are off to Virginia Beach for a few days on Saturday. Some folks have generously given us the time at their beach house. We are all really looking forward to getting away and being at the beach. May you all know how much God loves you and rejoice in His Son, our Savior's resurrection!

Love and blessings.
Carol, Tony, Chris, and Darcy

April 11, 2007

The nice long span between chemo really was a treat. VA beach was awesome. We all forgot how much we missed the sand and waves. And family and friends arrived for our Easter holiday. We are so fortunate and cherish all these special times with them. Chris had lots of energy and was able to really enjoy the festivities. Monday at clinic his blood counts were great. His ANC was 2290!! Monday was a long and hard day of three chemos, spinal tap, increased doses, and the lung breathing, yucky tasting stuff. He has been nauseous and very tired. But I think he is bouncing back quicker than before and we are all hopeful that he will be able to put in a few hours at school really soon. Darcy, along with a friend, is conducting the Leukemia & Lymphoma Penny Drive at her school this week. And she has been accepted into UVA's hospital intern volunteer role for the summer. Thank you all for your prayers. We love you and we feel those prayers. Our God is good.

Love,
Carol, Tony, Chris, and Darcy

April 21, 2007

Chris is doing great. His treatments went well on Thursday; his counts were all up as well. He did miss school on Thursday and Friday but has completed the math assignments and has just one more assignment in Lang. Arts to work on!!! His nausea seemed better. I think not having the spinal tap really helped. The next phase, which lasts approximately sixty days, is called Delayed Intensification. Chris starts this phase on the 3rd of May. It is supposed to be, as the name implies, Intense. But we know that it has an end and at the end, Chris will have his PICC line removed and begin the maintenance phase, which is supposed to be much easier. But Chris is a warrior and our God is so good! Thanks again for all the prayers, notes, support, and love. Enjoy the sunshine.

Love,
Carol, Tony, Chris, and Darcy

May 2, 2007

Chris has been doing great. Last week he put in a full week of school and continues to do the same this week. Tomorrow we head for clinic and begin the next phase. It includes four chemos, a spinal tap, and the yucky breathing stuff. This phase lasts fifty-seven days with chemo every day. So thank you for all your prayers and your prayers to come. We are truly being held up. Our Savior restores!!! Have a blessed day.

Love,
Carol, Tony, Chris, and Darcy

May 6, 2007

Chris started delayed intensification on Thursday and it proved to be INTENSE!! But it's Sunday a.m. and he is already up and playing video games! He has started eating again, thank God for Boost. Thursday will be the toughest day for the next few weeks, so we are all geared up and Chris is a strong warrior. God has equipped him for this battle and with your prayers he will be victorious. Darcy is at the beach in North Carolina with the youth group. We are grateful for any diversions she can experience during this stressful time. Again, thank you for your prayers. May God bless you all.

Love,
Carol, Tony, Chris, and Darcy

May 12, 2007

Chris is doing wonderfully!! Normally we need a wheelchair to get him to the car and last week he was vomiting for days. But God is so good. This week Chris walked out of clinic and experienced NO vomiting. He had some tiredness and stomach pain, but it's Saturday and he is doing great. He's gone for a short walk, is eating great, and even got himself caught up on schoolwork from the two days he missed this week. So, needless to say, God has given me an incredible mother's day gift. Thanks to all who have been praying for Chris and for our Wednesday home group lifting Chris and Darcy up in prayer. Thank You, God, for having such a tender and merciful heart.

Love and Blessings to all.
Carol, Tony, Chris, and Darcy

May 24, 2007

A quick update on Chris. His blood counts were unbelievably good today, with an ANC of over 7000!!! He is feeling really good. He was able to get his next round of heavy treatment pushed back so that his prom would be doable. So his next treatment will not be until Monday, June 4th. He has been working hard and having fun on the video he is making for the upcoming UVA oncology event on June 2nd. He is almost complete. He is caught up at school and it is nearly winding down. So again thank you for all your prayers and support.

We love you.
Carol, Tony, Chris, and Darcy

June 4, 2007

Well today was to be the start of the second half of delayed intensification but it has been delayed!! You need an ANC of 750 to begin and Chris's was 230. Quite a drop from the May 27th count of over 7000. They seemed surprised but these things happen. Apparently the chemo of the last round has had a delayed effect on his white blood cell count. So we are to bring in a blood sample on Thursday, in the hope that it has risen. They have tentatively scheduled the spinal tap (his eleventh) and the chemos for Friday. But we didn't, or Chris, get off scot-free. Anticipating the procedures caused hives and nausea on the way to the hospital. Despite meds, vomiting began. Increased anxiety arrived when Chris found out that the dreaded breathing procedure, which they usually do as he is coming out of sedation from a spinal tap, had to be performed today with no sedation. It produced more vomiting, nausea, and ended with a splotchy rash. Chris is becoming known as the "rash kid" at clinic. That's why he has to do the breathing procedure rather than take a simple pill to ward off lung infections, because of allergic reactions. But he is feeling better as I write and we are all going to settle in to a movie night. He's hoping to go to school tomorrow so he can see friends before the school year officially ends on Friday. Please pray that this breathing thing goes better as he faces about thirty-five more rounds of it before his chemo ends approximately three years from now. Also, we ask for prayers that Chris's counts go up so he can resume his therapy on Friday. Having his Nana here has been a blessing to all of us. Additional blessings, Darcy ended her school year receiving three academic awards of excellence and [sic] Chris is complete in all subjects and had lots of fun at his prom. God has definitely been holding us in the palm of His hand. And I am sure this delay will only strengthen Chris prior to going into his next battle. God is good. May you feel His blessings in your lives this week.

Love,
Carol, Tony, Chris, and Darcy

June 8, 2007

Well, Chris's counts continue to stay too low to begin the next phase. They barely climbed, his ANC is still in the 230 range. It needs to be above 750 to start. The ANC is the Absolute Neutrophil Count and is based on the amount of white blood cells ready to do battle. Unlike platelets and red blood cells, you cannot transfuse white blood cells. The white blood cells just have to come up on their own. This week has also been the HIVE week. The anticipatory hives he had last week at clinic turned out to be an allergic reaction. They have continued all week but thankfully have finally abated. So we are in a holding pattern. We are scheduled to bring in a blood sample next Wednesday and if the counts are good, Thursday will be a long day at clinic, with a spinal tap and four chemos. We'll keep you posted. For now we will enjoy this break and we pray you will all have a break in your hectic lives to enjoy!!! God is GOOOOOD!!!

Love,
Carol, Tony, Chris, and Darcy

June 19, 2007

Sorry for the delayed update on Chris. He did start the next phase on Thursday, the 14th. He handled the spinal tap and chemos well. He did experience vomiting and nausea for the first three days. Nausea has persisted but not with such a vengeance. Today has been stomach cramping but we seem to have gotten him comfortable for now. He will start the second half of this phase on Thursday, the 21st. It will be his twelfth spinal tap with three chemos. We will continue to give chemo at home through his IV, through Sunday. Oral chemo will continue through next Wednesday, the 27th. Then he gets a rest till his counts build up again. We are anticipating some blood transfusions in the next few weeks as his counts will continue to drop as a result of the cumulative effects of the drugs. The hospital has warned us to anticipate a hospital stay, as it is quite common during this phase. So our prayers are to avoid the hospital stay, and for Chris to stay emotionally, spiritually, and physically strong, putting his trust in the Lord. We are thankful for how our Lord has been so faithful and we thank Him in advance for taking Chris through this phase. Soon Chris will be able to have his PICC line removed (Hooray!!) and although the treatment continues it is supposed to be very tolerable. Darcy started her intern volunteer position at UVA yesterday and loved it. She is working today in the adult oncology floor. She will be rotating through four different roles. Wednesday she leaves for a four-day field hockey camp at William & Mary. She has a busy summer ahead of her. Nana has remained with us, which is such a blessing. It will be very hard to say goodbye. We are so thankful for your prayers. We never feel like we are doing it alone. God is so good and His army is awesome. Thank you all.

Blessings and Love,
Carol, Tony, Chris, and Darcy

June 25, 2007

Good News. Chris has been handling things really well. Thank You, Lord!!! He is done with the harshest of the chemos for this phase. His blood counts, however, are creeping down. His platelets dropped to 40 and his hemoglobin dropped to 11. They transfuse at 20 and 8 respectively. So right now we are in a watch and see situation. He does go back for a shot of Vincristine (chemo) and the breathing meds to ward off lung infections on Thursday. His friend Marcus is headed over to hang out with him for a while today. Life gets so routine when your activity level is so low. His Nana has been such good medicine but she will be headed to MD and then on to NJ on Saturday. We will miss her terribly. Darcy had a great time at William & Mary's field hockey clinic. Tony completed a mini triathlon on Sunday in under two hours. So all is well at the Alimenti household. We thank you for your prayers and praise Our Lord for His faithful, loving watch over all His children.

Love,
Carol, Tony, Chris, and Darcy

June 28, 2007

I feel such hesitancy in updating tonight but I am trying to trust God and not be fearful. Chris had a seizure on Tuesday. We went by ambulance to the hospital and he was discharged late Wednesday night. It was really scary. But he is doing much better now. This round of chemo is very hard and just takes him down. There are blessings. They suspected he might have suffered a stroke but the

MRI revealed no abnormalities. Second blessing, when he hit his head, his platelets were dangerously low—"feet on the ground rule" (clotting problems), but the CAT scan was fine. Thank You, Jesus. So all in all we have lots to be thankful for. They have given him two platelet and one red blood cell transfusion. Today was a long hospital day. Coupled with the transfusions, he received chemo and the "yucky" breathing stuff. He's still nauseous but we are diligently administering the anti-nausea meds. He is lying on the couch peacefully watching a John Wayne flick. No more chemo till next Thursday. His counts will continue to drop so we will be bringing blood samples in on Monday. Thank you all for your prayers.

Love,
Carol, Tony, Chris, and Darcy

July 5, 2007

Chris had his last round of chemo today for this final phase. His blood counts are coming up, so there were no transfusions needed!!! His white blood counts are very low but they are also showing signs of moving upward. He is tired and pretty much vegged out all day. We are hopeful that tomorrow he will have more energy. We bring in a sample of his blood on the 9th to check how his counts are doing. It is not till the 16th that he is scheduled for his next clinic visit. So a nice long stretch. On the 16th he will begin the Maintenance phase which will end 3 years from this past April (April 2010). It will consist of repeated ninety day cycles. Oral chemo will be administered daily. The 16th will include a spinal tap w/chemo, an IV chemo push, and two oral chemos. But the good news is, they will remove his PICC line. We are continually reassured that although it doesn't look easy, it is a lot more tolerable than what he has been through. And having his PICC line out will be quite freeing. It has placed restrictions on his activities and has demanded much daily maintenance, Tony has done an excellent job at keeping infection free. So all in all, we are psyched!!! Chris has been quite the warrior. Our family continues to grow closer and we all continue to be awed at our

Lord's faithfulness in taking us through this journey. Thank you for being a part of our lives and helping us through Chris's illness. Our family will be forever thankful.

Blessings,
Carol, Tony, Chris, and Darcy

July 12, 2007

Chris is presently playing X-Box and just hanging out. He did make it to the gym with Tony today for a light workout. He had a long hospital day on Monday. We were there for twelve hours. Chris received 3 units of blood and has been quite peppy since. His white count was still in the critical range but we are praying that by Monday the 16th all his counts will have risen and he can begin the Maintenance Phase. Darcy is loving her hospital volunteering but moaning through her field hockey conditioning. Lots of running!! She leaves on Saturday for a week of babysitting and vacationing with my sister Anne and her family in Kure Island, NC. Hope you are all enjoying your summer and remember to stop by if you are in our area.

Love and blessings,
Carol, Tony, Chris, and Darcy

July 16, 2007

Chris had his clinic visit today. All his blood counts were up. Thank You, Lord. In fact, his platelets were normal, his white blood cells went from 0.2 to 2.58, a low number but no longer a critical one. His red blood count went to 13.5, which is 0.5 shy of normal!!! Chris had his thirteenth spinal tap and four types of chemo today. He was vomiting and nauseous but is presently resting comfortably. He also had to have his yucky breathing stuff to ward off lung infections. But the upside of the day was the removal of his PICC line. Tony is planning some kind of cremation ceremony for his PICC line to mark this milestone. Thankfully, Chris doesn't return to the clinic until 8/13. From now until the next clinic all his chemos will be administered orally on a daily basis. Lots of pills but no hospital, no PICC line, and a much more tolerable regime. We are team captains for "Light the Night," a fund raising walk for the Leukemia & Lymphoma Society. The walk takes place in Charlottesville on October 11th. If you are interested in joining our walking team or wish to donate to the cause, please feel free to visit our website: http://www.active.com/donate/ ltnRichmo/2134_alimenti. We are forever grateful for the grace that God extends to us each and every day. His grace is sufficient. Thanks for your prayers, love, and support.

Love and Blessings,
Carol, Tony, Chris, and Darcy

July 26, 2007

Chris is doing great!!! Maintenance is proving to be a more tolerable regime. On Tuesday I loaded the trunk with all the medical supplies we no longer needed now that his PICC line was removed. It was such a blessing to reach this milestone. I have whined about our medical out of pocket expenses but as I wheeled the cart of supplies to clinic I realized how fortunate we are to have insurance. The nurses all helped with the unloading happily, knowing that they would be able to pass these supplies on to families in need. We all enjoyed having Tony's folks here for the weekend. Visitors are such good medicine. Chris was able to hang out last night at a friend's.

Love,
Carol, Tony, Chris, and Darcy

August 13, 2007

Well the big clinic day came. Chris was really anxious but he made it through his fourteenth spinal tap and the receiving of four chemos today. They are skipping the "yucky" breathing stuff and he will, by choice, be taking a liquid med every day to ward off lung infections. Not quite sure yet how that will all play out. He has had a lot of vomiting and nausea and just seems really wiped.

But by tomorrow he will be feeling better and by Wednesday he'll be that much stronger. Pat, his nurse today and Ginger and Gwen, the other nurses, were, as usual, just wonderful. They show such compassion and love. Our prayers for now are that the chemo does its thing and quickly moves through him, that his vomiting stops and he experiences no additional side effects. It's so hard because he has such a long road ahead but one step at a time is all we can do. Thank you for your prayers. Our God is good and He loves us all dearly.

Love and blessings,
Carol, Tony, Chris, and Darcy

August 16, 2007

It's Thursday a.m. and Chris is feeling great. Thank You, Lord, for such a speedy rebound and for all the prayers offered to You in Chris's name. Tony and Chris are headed on Saturday to see the Mets in DC against the Nationals. Chris is so excited, he is an avid Mets fan. He even has his mom watching and cheering them on! Darcy was chosen to participate in her high school's Women's Advanced Chorale. She is also very busy with her field hockey practices. She ended her hospital volunteer position receiving the "Above & Beyond" Award. School starts next Wednesday, the 22nd. Not being a warm weather fan, I am gladly looking forward to autumn. Tony and I are doing well and we all thank you for your faithful support.

Love and God Bless,
Carol, Tony, Chris, and Darcy

September 7, 2007

Clinic time is nearing, Monday the 10th, and this always creates anxiety for Chris. Also, he has been experiencing lots of nausea, several bouts of vomiting, and fatigue. Unfortunately, all of this goes with the territory but he is well aware that this is his life for the next several years. Our prayer requests at this time are for Chris to experience minimal side effects, for endurance and stamina for the long haul, for Our Lord's calming spirit to grow within him. On the upside, he is enjoying school and being with friends. In addition, he has started an acting for film class, which is really exciting him. Darcy has quite the academic load as well as juggling field hockey. We are praying she does not stress over it. We are all learning through this experience that life should be enjoyed, laughter is good for the soul, to follow our passions and love one another. Thanks for your prayers and support.

Sending you all our love,
Carol, Tony, Chris, and Darcy

September 15, 2007

This week was a bit rocky but, thankfully, it is closing on an upbeat. The nausea, vomiting, and fatigue all turned out to be connected with the liver. Chris went into a liver overload, normal range 0.3 to 1.2. Chris's bilirubin was 5.5, but as of Thursday it was, thankfully, down to 2.8. They gave him several bags of saline to help flush things through and have halted all chemotherapy till his counts normalize. Chris was at clinic 3 times this week and is scheduled for a visit on Monday. Because he no longer has a PICC line they have to set up an IV line on each visit. Ouch!! The blessings—no permanent liver damage and his body is getting a chance to rest. In addition, Chris made it to school two full days and part of a third day! Tony really carried the burden as I connected with family in NJ/NY from Tuesday to Friday. Tony's folks are headed here on Sunday for a visit. We are so thankful for the time we get to spend with family and friends. We hope that you all enjoy this lovely autumn weather and thank you all for your continued prayers and support.

Love,
Carol, Tony, Chris, and Darcy

September 24, 2007

It's Monday and we spent, to Chris's chagrin, four hours at clinic. The long and short is his counts are still not right. So it continues to be a wait and see policy, with a return to clinic on Thursday. The good news is he hasn't been getting chemo. The bad news is he soon will!! But he had a great birthday weekend and even went to the UVA football game, which they won. So I will keep you posted and thanks again for hanging in there with us.

Love,
Carol, Tony, Chris, and Darcy

September 28, 2007

We need prayer. Chris's ANC, which is a measure of white blood cells available to fight off infection has continued to drop, currently at 94. On Monday at 8 a.m. we will head back to clinic. If his blood work is still off, they have a bone marrow test scheduled for 9 a.m. They are looking to see if Chris has relapsed and the leukemia is back. Please keep Chris in your prayers this weekend. We are not going to go into detail with Chris and Darcy this weekend regarding the doctor's suspicions. Chris is planning to attend a UVA football game on Saturday night with Tony. We will be doing as much fun stuff as possible. So if you see either of them, mum's the word. Just pray. May we all enjoy this weekend and give thanks to our Maker.

Love and God Bless,
Carol, Tony, Chris, and Darcy

October 1, 2007

We just received notice—Chris's bone marrow test was negative for leukemia—he has **not** had a relapse!!!!!! Thank You, Lord, and thank you all for keeping Chris in your prayers the last few days. God is good!

God bless,
Carol, Tony, Chris, and Darcy

October 4, 2007

Chris was at clinic today for blood work. Some of you have asked, "Have his counts come up?" The answer is, "Very slowly." His ANC today was 366. In order to take Methotrexate and/or

Mercaptopurine he needs to have an ANC of 750 or greater. They also performed a special test, but will take several weeks to get the results back. The test will tell if Chris has a genetically low production of an enzyme needed to metabolize Mercaptopurine. That would explain the liver toxicity issue and his suppressed ANC. Based on that test and its resulting number they will have to lower the overall doses Chris receives and closely monitor his liver functions. Please pray for discernment for the doctors and that lowering the dosages will in no way compromise the effectiveness of Chris's treatment. Thanks for all your prayers and continued support.

God Bless,
Carol, Tony, Chris, and Darcy

October 8, 2007

Lots of prayer and **Thank You, God**, Chris's counts came up. His ANC this morning was 1003! He had a full day at clinic. He received his fifteenth spinal tap with Methotrexate, Vincristine, the yucky breathing stuff, and a flu shot. He handled everything great. Tonight he will begin the 6MP at half dose and his five-day round of steroids. We head back to the clinic next Monday to check how his blood counts and liver are handling the restart of his chemo. It will still be another week or so for the results on the enzyme test. Right now he is sleeping on the couch. Pray he wakes refreshed. Tomorrow at 7:30 a.m. the local TV news station, Channel 29, arrives to interview him. It will air on the 11th to promote the Leukemia & Lymphoma Society "Light the Night Walk." So all you locals watch for his debut. Thanks again for all your love and support. And thanks to Greg for the sailing diversion excursion on Sunday.

Love,
Carol, Tony, Chris, and Darcy

October 12, 2007

The "Light the Night" walk for the Leukemia & Lymphoma Society last night went well. Thanks to all for your prayers and support. For a short time, you can go to the URL below and see Chris and Darcy's interview

106

with the NBC Channel 29 reporters. Living with Leukemia: Chris's Story http://www.nbc29com/Global/story.asp?s=7199515. Hope all is well with you.

God Bless,
Tony, Carol, Chris, and Darcy

October 18, 2007

A quick update. Chris's counts were great on Monday. The enzyme test was performed incorrectly, so we are now waiting on a new test result. This test will determine if he genetically lacks sufficient TPMT enzymes to properly metabolize a chemo drug he takes every day for the next two and a half years. They lowered the amount on Monday by fifty percent. This coming Monday he returns to the clinic to recheck blood, specifically his bilirubin, to check for liver toxicity. We have a French exchange student with us and my mom. We are all enjoying their visits. Darcy's field hockey ended the season undefeated and unscored upon. Next Monday is the district championship game. Her choral performance, which Chris taped for us, was wonderful. We were at the Leukemia Walk. The turnout was great, over sixty grand was raised for research! Hope you all were able to view the kids' interviews on our local TV station. Have a wonderful day. Bon jour!!!

Love and God Bless,
Carol, Tony, Chris, and Darcy

October 23, 2007

Chris's counts were great. The bilirubin moved up slightly but is still just within the normal range. They are keeping the 6MP drugs at fifty percent and we are still waiting for the enzyme test results. He is at school and although Mondays are a big chemo night, he is doing great. Darcy's team won the final championship game!! We all continue to feel blessed by all your love and support. May you all walk in God's love and peace.

Carol, Tony, Chris, and Darcy

November 17, 2007

Chris has been doing great!! It turned out that he has a normal enzyme level to properly metabolize the chemo. They now feel he must have had some type of virus to explain the liver toxicity issue??? He will be rechecked on the 19th and watched but so far so good! He did suffer some stomach discomfort from the last heavy round but even for that we seem to be understanding what do to minimize the discomfort. So we are off to my niece's in Manassas for Thanksgiving Day and then on to Tony's folks in PA for a few days. We are all looking forward to spending the holidays with family. We have so much to be thankful for. This Wednesday marks the one-year anniversary of Chris's diagnosis. We spent last Thanksgiving in a hospital. But when I look back on this year, I clearly see God's grace and His mercy in our lives. And how much we have been blessed with family, friends, finances, hospital, medical staff, love, and most importantly, prayer. Thank you all!!! Happy Thanksgiving!

Love,
Carol, Tony, Chris, and Darcy

December 11, 2007

Just a quick update to let you know that Chris is doing great! Thank you all for the prayers, love, and support you have showered us with this past year. As my close friend, Donna, said, "Carol, do you realize that every prayer request you asked was answered?" Our God is so faithful. Even in our times of trials, even when we are unaware, God is forever merciful. May we all go through this holiday season mindful of His blessings, His mercy, and His grace. Merry Christmas.

Love,
Carol, Tony, Chris, and Darcy

January 4, 2008

Happy New Year!!! Chris had his eighteenth spinal tap and all sorts of chemos plus the yucky breathing stuff yesterday. He walked out of the clinic, spent the rest of the night on the couch, and this a.m. was up and arrived at his school about ten minutes late!!! Thank You, Lord for taking all of us by Your hand as we walk, crawl, and sometimes run through our life journey. Please keep another C'ville family and young girl in your prayers as they now face very similar circumstances. Chris does have a low platelet and an elevated bilirubin count. Next Thursday he will go in to the clinic to have his counts rechecked. So please pray for normalized counts. Thank You, Lord, for all the good You have brought to us as a family and to each of us individually over the course of this past year. May we continue to keep You utmost in our lives. Thank You, Lord, for Your mercy and grace. And thank You, Lord, for all the wonderful family and friends You have placed in our lives. God Bless you all!

Carol, Tony, Chris, and Darcy

January 17, 2008

I wanted to give you a quick update on Chris's labs. He went in on Thursday, the 10th, and the bilirubin was elevated but the platelets had improved. So they had him go in today, the 17th, and the bilirubin had dropped (which is good news) but it is still out of the normal range. But now his platelets dropped (which is not what they want). So the long and short of it is we are headed back to clinic on Monday, the 21st, for more lab work. No more PICC lines so lots of needle sticking. Chris never complains about being stuck, thank God! We received some snow and the kids were home today and will be home tomorrow and have a scheduled day off on Monday. So it's lots of hot chocolate and hanging around. Hope you are all enjoying the New Year!

Love,
Carol, Tony, Chris, and Darcy

January 23, 2008
New lab results from Monday, the 21st. Chris's bilirubin is normal and his platelets are up (at 100), also a good thing. His white blood

count, Neutrophil counts are down. This means high risk of infection due to low defense fighter availability. But the rainbow is no chemo till rechecks on Monday. They don't want to further suppress his counts and they want to give him time to recover. So we all like these little breaks in the protocol. All in all, Chris is feeling good and doing lots and lots of hand sanitizing. Thanks for all your prayers.

Love,
Carol, Tony, Chris, and Darcy

February 4, 2008

Last Monday Chris received his spinal tap w/the Methotrexate, Vincristine, and started the steroids. His counts were too low so they stopped the MP6. We returned on Thursday and his counts came up so they started his MP6 at fifty percent and tonight he will take his Methotrexate at fifty percent. They plan to increase both very slowly and continually check his counts. Our prayer request at this time is for Chris's lymphocyte counts to rise to the normal range. Chris is slow to rebuild white blood cells after his chemo, therefore there have been these continual disruptions in his protocol. Thankfully, Chris has been in good spirits. The Giants winning last night was a real plus!! Family and friends and lots of laughter continue to be the best Rx. Thanks for your prayers and may you all feel God's blessings today.

Love,
Carol, Tony, Chris, and Darcy

February 15, 2008

Chris had his blood work yesterday. His counts stayed about the same, dropped slightly, so they are increasing his chemo to seventy-five percent. We head back to clinic on Monday, the 25th. Overall, he has been in good spirits. We continue to thank you all for your prayers and support.

Love and God Bless,
Carol, Tony, Chris, and Darcy

March 11, 2008

Things have been going really well. Chris's counts were up and they increased his Methotrexate to 100 percent—fifteen pills taken every Monday. They still have his 6MP at seventy-five percent, which is taken daily. This Tuesday a.m. he is already off to school. Driving solo! And left with a big smile on his face. Chris is also completely weaned off of his seizure meds, which means six less pills a day!!! Thank You, God, and thank you all who continue to lift our family up in prayer. May you all feel His peace and joy in your lives this week. Darcy is back and forth to the doctors, trying to understand and help some of her hormonal/ thyroid issues which have been plaguing her.

April 25, 2008

It's been a while since I have updated you folks. Things have been going really well. We spent six days visiting my family at different locations throughout Florida for the spring break. It was great to see everyone. We also made it up to Scranton, PA, for Easter with all of Tony's family. Chris did have clinic on Monday, which turned out to be a roller coaster of a day. But it all ended in praises. His blood showed atypical cells and he has had a declining platelet level for the last three months. He was also very neutropenic (low white blood count). They performed a bone marrow test to make sure he had not relapsed. We had the good news by 4:30 p.m., no leukemia was present. Chris probably had a bug. Because his counts are low they have suspended his MP6 which he takes daily and until they come up, no Methotrexate as well. He goes back to clinic on Monday to get checked out. But he looks great and is out with a buddy tonight. So he gets a little break from some of the chemo, which he really likes! Darcy is a busy, busy girl with rehearsals till late for the school play, *Once Upon a Mattress*. Tony and I are doing good, enjoying one of our favorite seasons, as we both love to garden. We pray that you are all doing well and also enjoying God's spring extravaganza!

God bless,
Carol, Tony, Chris, and Darcy

May 14, 2008

I felt a strong need to shout THANK YOU!!! Chris had remained off chemo due to low, low counts that were creeping up ever so slowly for the last 3 weeks. Chris was beginning to allow the word relapse to sink into his thoughts. But our Great Physician took his ANC (absolute Neutrophil) count of May 8th @ 220 and miraculously raised it by May 12th to **2490**. More than a tenfold increase in four days!! It needed to come up to at least 500 to restart the chemo. Thank You, Lord, and thank you all for keeping Chris in your prayers. Our God is a God of miracles.

Love and God Bless,
Carol, Tony, Chris, and Darcy

November 30, 2008

Dear friends and family,
It has been a while since we have written. Chris has been doing great. He has made it through two years of treatment. November 21st was his anniversary. He still has another one and a half years to complete his protocol but he looks great, is working at Carmike movie theater, completing his senior year of high school, doing an acting internship, and both he & Darcy just got parts in the school's spring musical *Urinetown*. Also Chris's Make-a-Wish happened, so check out the photos of the Alimentis & Robin Williams. One week prior to Chris's anniversary Tony took me, Carol, over to the ER due to a persistent back pain. I was operated on on 11/17 to remove an egg-sized tumor that had compressed my spinal cord to a ribbon. Numerous doctors acclaimed the miracle that I was not paralyzed. But it didn't stop there. Chris is okay with my sharing his site. He does have a spinal tap and a long treatment day this Monday. I will simultaneously visit a UVA surgeon. They have found that I have an advanced stage IV case of leiomyosarcoma. Radiation will begin first, followed by chemo and then possibly additional surgeries. My older sister, Annie, whom I called from the ER has spent the last two weeks being our guardian angel. My mom, the family ROCK, is still with us and is sitting by my side while I write this. My other siblings are in Florida, Joy and Michael,

and they are very anxious about coming to help. Being at a distance is so hard. Tony and Darcy are trying to "maintain" as we deal with a second cancer in two years' time. There is a second tumor on my spine at T7, which has caused a fracture at that site. They will be making a body cast so I lay perfectly still as they do some high dose treatments to that site. The operated site at T11 will be radiated after that for two weeks. The tumor has eaten into the bone at that site. The chemo is a protocol developed at Sloan-Kettering. The other tumors are in the liver (two), kidney, and spleen. Pray they can shrink the tumors trough the radiation. I'll keep you updated on the progress. We do appreciate all your prayers and the meals and caring. Today the reality for me seems to be seeping in and the burden it will place on my family. Please pray that can be lifted.

Love,
Carol, Tony, Chris, and Darcy

November 30, 2008

Check out the link below to view Chris's movie:

Live, Laugh, Love, Part 1 link: http://www.youtube.com/watch?v=OoGAl6kEYCs

LLL part 2 link: http://www.youtube.com/watch?v=bIV8NlppLBE
Chris's home page: http://home.comcast.net/~paintballchris98/site/

December 2, 2008

Thank you all for your notes and prayers. Chris had his 26th, I think, spinal tap yesterday. He did great, he is my hero. Went to school today and to acting class tonight. Tony & I met w/ neurosurgery yesterday and my incision was glued and looks great. Today we met with radiation. A body cast was started, it takes some time to form, my radiation will start on the two spots on my spine on the 15th. My oncologist is requesting a consult w/ Sloan-Kettering. At first they said four weeks but he is trying to go through the dept. chair and get it moved up. So Tony and I will be making a quick run to

NYC. Fortunately, insurance will cover even our travel, but due to physical therapy and other appointments it will not allow time to visit w/ our friends & family. S-K has done the most on this cancer and seeing as it is so rare and advanced, they really would like me to see if a clinical trial they offer might be the best option. All the treatments can occur at UVA, they do this kind of thing all the time. So pray all the arrangements can go smoothly. Thank you again for two years of support and love. And we feel so blessed by "you all" (a little southern gal for y'all).

Love and God bless,
Carol, Tony, Chris, and Darcy

December 12, 2008

Chris is doing great. He is at his job at the movie theater tonight. He still is very stuffy. Tony, Darcy, and I met with oncology today. It was a unanimous decision on the part of the doctors to get a consult from Sloan-Kettering. All my info (slides, scans, pathology reports) will be sent ahead of time for the doctors to review. We will be in New York City on January 13th. Radiation begins on my spine on Monday and will last through the first of the year. My chemo is tentatively scheduled for when we return from NYC dependent on their findings. Please pray that the radiation melts away the tumors on my spine. Also, that I experience minimal side effects. And that Chris gets over the stuffy nose. Thanks for all your support, concern, and prayers!

Love and God Bless,
Carol, Tony, Chris, Darcy, and Nana

December 15, 2008

Thank you all for the prayers. Radiation went well and I am headed back there tomorrow. Chris took his Methotrexate today and is making it through it. Thanks for everything.

Love,
The Alimentis

December 18, 2008

I [Carol] finished up the three-day special radiation zap to the T7 tumor on my spine. Today I had the first of ten zaps to my T11 spot. I lie in my pod (cast) and envision I am being held in God's everlasting arms, the shelter of His wings. I envision the radiation as His healing light attacking all the tumors and cancer cells. It has been a very peaceful experience so far. Fatigue is all I have experienced so far and everyone should experience the joy of napping!!! Chris was busy Christmas shopping and is now wrapping presents. He is definitely getting into the spirit. Darcy is studying for her last two exams!!!! I know she is very anxious to get into the holiday spirit and bake cookies. Tony turns fifty-four tomorrow. So we have some celebrating to do. Thank you all for your prayers.

Love,
Carol, Tony, Chris, and Darcy

January 7, 2009

Sorry for the delay in updating this journal. Chris is doing well, a little sick after they increased his MTX, but he bounces back. He is getting closer to the end of his treatment (April 2010 ~ 1.3 yrs to go!!). Carol finished her radiation (3 on T7 and 10 on T11) Jan 2nd. She is doing well, very tired as expected but no apparent burns or severe side effects. We met with the surgeon yesterday, and things are progressing. We'll meet with him again in six weeks. It takes a couple of months to determine the radiation's effect. We are scheduled for testing this Friday to get a picture as to how/where the tumors are versus their state in November. Pray that they haven't grown and have even shrunk. We go to Sloan-Kettering next week for the consult. Pray that what they state is implementable here @ UVA and whatever the chemo protocol is, that it works with minimal side effects. We thank you for all your prayers and support over the past years and months. It is through those prayers that we have been sustained.

Thanks and God Bless,
Carol, Tony, Chris, & Darcy

January 9, 2009

Carol had a CAT scan today to mark the status of the tumors since they were last checked in November. This is in prep for our trip to NYC on Monday and the start of chemo on TH. Have I captured your interest in the results? Well, we are truly blessed, thanks for your prayers, and God has blessed us with some grace and good news. The tumors have not changed in size nor have any new tumors appeared. In fact, the tumor in the spleen appears to be an accumulation of blood processing through it. (I'll leave it to the doctors in the reading list to provide a more accurate description). The tumor in the lung is possibly a calcification. The two in the spine (well, now one since the surgery) the two in the liver and the one in the kidney have not grown nor multiplied. There was a note about another in the pelvic region, but since the report indicated that it hadn't changed either since the last reading, we probably didn't remember there was one there. In any case, this is good news. This provides a nonmoving target for the chemo and radiation to perform their work. We are relieved and Carol's spirit is renewed! Albeit a slow and arduous path, we are seeing and living via the support of grace through the intercession of friends and family. There is still a long way to go, but living each day in relationship with God and with those whom God placed in our paths is a real blessing for which we are ever thankful. So, we will enjoy this news and build up strength for the next step. Please continue to "stand strong" and continue in prayer for our travel to/from NYC and the resultant protocol direction. We are hoping all administration of the chemo can be done in UVA so as to keep the family together as Chris has one year and four months and counting left on his protocol @ UVA. We give thanks to you all and also for the researchers, doctors, nurses, technicians, and staff who have dedicated themselves to being God's healing vessels. May Christ's peace be with you always.

Carol, Tony, Chris, and Darcy

January 15, 2009

Thanks so much for your prayers. Our NYC trip to S/K went very well, the doctors suggested we start with a different chemo (Doxil) that is supposed to have less of a harsh effect. We were able to meet with some friends, and it turned out to be a great trip! Many blessings and healing. Today, we went to the hospital @ 10 to start the process, Carol got a (MUGA scan?) to baseline her heart and ensure it is strong enough. We met with the Dr. to review everything and start the Doxil. We were very optimistic with the process and the steps agreed upon. Carol started receiving some pre-chemo drugs to minimize the irritation of the chemo and did develop some side effects. They had to back off a little and dilute with saline. She started to feel better. They then administered the Doxil and then she started to experience all the side effects listed in the chart for allergic reactions, that only happens in 10 percent of the population. The team immediately stopped the chemo and worked hard and got things under control. She is stable and at home now. They plan to try again next TH, with some other pre-drugs to minimize the side effects. She is going to start taking those ~ thirteen hours before treatment. So, again, thanks for your prayers, we have some days that appear like all is well and others that remind us of how much we are dependent on God's will. So pray that God is gentle with us and that we can feel the grace that He bestowed on us through NYC when we are in the midst of other trials. Carol read a passage the other day: "tears are the Holy Spirit's means of tenderizing our hearts." We are all challenged, may God bless us all. May Christ's peace be with you.

Carol, Tony, Chris, and Darcy

January 22, 2009

I'll try this again. CaringBridge locked up right as I [Tony] was saving it. . . . Carol started the Doxil this morning after some preventative Dex, Benadryl last night at 8:30, 2:30, and 8:30 this morning. Then in the clinic at 9:30 she got some more Dex/Benadryl as well as some Ativan, then a dextrose flush before the Doxil was administered. Initially the Doxil was given in a slow and diluted manner. After some initial pains that eventually subsided, they were able to go up to full dosage until about half the bag was delivered. Then around 3, she started developing a rash that spread over her body. They stopped the Doxil immediately and then administered some more Benadryl and Dexamethasone. They got the allergic reaction under control and we were home by 5. We see the Dr. tomorrow morning to follow up on the rash and review what the next steps will be in terms of treatment, drugs, etc. They can't do the Doxil anymore as she has exhibited a full allergic response, and since she received about half a normal dosage, they have to wait a couple of weeks before starting another drug. She will most likely start exhibiting the chemo side effects but possibly not bringing her counts down too low. However, blood tests etc. will be done to determine the extent of the impact. We will know more tomorrow as to the next steps. Thanks to the doctors and nurses who are doing a great job with a challenging case. Thanks again for your prayers, support, and love. It is through this support that we are being upheld. It's those requests that the peace of God is protecting our hearts as we walk through this valley. Thank you and God Bless you, too.

Carol, Tony, Chris, and Darcy

February 1, 2009

I haven't written in quite a while. Tony has been doing a great job of keeping folks updated. But I am feeling much better and just wanted to thank you for all your prayers. Praises that our worst fears of having to receive treatment in NYC was squelched. Thankfully we are all comfortably at home, with a fifteen-minute drive, at most, to a great hospital. My oncologist is a wonderful young, dedicated doctor, who called us every day while we were in NYC. Chris's Monday clinic did reveal a higher than normal bilirubin level but not high enough to suspend treatments. He just left for a day of work and then he is planning to get together w/friends for Super Bowl. Both Darcy and Chris are busy w/play practices for *Urinetown*. I am finally coming off a long steroid regime. I have a whole new understanding of Chris having to receive mega steroids every fourth week. Your legs feel so heavy and climbing a flight of stairs is quite a feat. The how to proceed next regarding my protocol is in an iffy state at this time. They discussed many options but until rescanning in about two weeks nothing is set in stone. They are thinking that this upcoming week is when my blood counts will drop. So far I haven't experienced much, aside from the allergic reaction, from the chemo, so who knows. Prayers for Chris and his continued perseverance as he gets closer to his one-year countdown for completion. Prayers that my tumors are shrinking. I do feel that the one in my liver has already shrunk significantly. Prayers for our caretakers, Tony and Darcy, that they do not lose faith and hope. Prayers for increased laughter and joy to permeate our household. And prayers for my mom who is experiencing a health issue at this time. We again thank you for lifting us up in prayer and we pray that you will all be blessed and experience God's grace and mercy in your lives.

Love,
Carol, Tony, Chris, and Darcy

February 8, 2009

A quick update on the Alimenti household. My mom's surgery went well and thankfully they did not find a tumor in her kidney. The bleeding is still an unknown and they want to do more investigating. Chris just got back from the ER and he has the flu. Both my mom and I are being put on preventative meds. It is supposed to be a highly contagious strain, despite us all receiving flu shots. I am feeling really healthy and it will be at least a week and a half to two weeks before I receive another try at chemo. My sister has been here and will go w/me to take mom to two doctor appointments tomorrow. So we are quite a household! But we feel very blessed and strong in our knowledge that God is good and God heals. Thank you all for your prayers and we pray blessings for you and yours.

Love,
Carol, Tony, Chris, Darcy, Nana, and Oscar (arf)

February 10, 2009

Prayers for Chris. We made another ER visit last night w/Chris. The flu has really hit him hard and his liver functions went haywire. He rec'd 3 bags of fluids and we made it back home at 3 a.m. He has to be closely watched and thankfully his chemo has been temporarily suspended. So please keep him in your prayers for a speedy recovery. Thanks for loving on us. Pray blessings on you all.

Love,
the Alimentis

February 11, 2009

Chris was seen today at the hospital; he has a double ear infection. Thankfully the chest X-ray was normal! He was able to keep down some broth, and yogurt. He lost five pounds and if you know Chris, you know that he's a pretty skinny guy. He's resting lots and drinking fluids like crazy. Hope and pray none of you experience this yucky flu. One school in our area has closed due to the high incidence of the flu. Thanks again for your prayers.

God Bless,
the Alimentis

February 15, 2009

Chris is doing better. Still coughing but has started to keep down solids. His chemo has been suspended since Monday. We will check w/his doctors tomorrow and see how to proceed. I will be having a CAT scan on Thursday and the doctors will determine how to proceed on my chemo based on those results. I will also be having a spinal X-ray on Tuesday to see how the old spine is doing. My mom will have ultrasounds, CAT scan, and PET scan this week as well. So it is the testing week at the Alimentis. Praises that Chris is doing better and prayers that all our test results come back with the best possible outcomes. Also Tony's brother has been experiencing health problems but is now, thankfully, at home resting. Prayers that he will experience full healing. Thank you to all our prayer warriors for your continued dedication. May you all experience a blessed day.

Love and God bless,
the Alimentis

February 20, 2009

Test updates and praise outcomes! Chris has been back to work, school, and his play practice. A little stuffy but totally on the mend. He started back on his chemo regimen and seems to be handling it well. He has a spinal tap and a big clinic day on Monday but all in all, he is doing great. My mom's PET scan & CAT scan found, thankfully, NO problems!! She does need to follow up next Thursday for a surgical consult on suspicious breast cysts that they have been following. They told her to be prepared for a biopsy to be performed. My doctor just called and my scans showed no new tumors and only a very slight increase in existing tumor size. He will be scheduling my infusion for next week but wants to run it past the dept. head on Monday to get his take on the protocol he plans to start me on. So we are thankful that the cancer is not progressing at a rapid rate, thankful that we live so close to a wonderful hospital, thankful that we have great doctors working on our cases, and thankful that there are drugs to fight our cancers. And thankful to all of you who continue to pray for our healing and our family's strength to handle the battles. As the apostle Paul wrote to the Philippians, "I can do everything through Him who gives me strength." Paul then adds, "Yet it was good of you to share in my troubles." That scripture sums it up for us at this time. Thanks for sharing in our troubles.

Love and God bless,
the Alimentis

March 1, 2009

Today most of us on the east coast are bracing for a snowstorm. I guess I rushed the purchase of pansies last week. I am so looking forward to spring. Last week Chris had a rough round with his spinal tap. It took multiple tries and has resulted in a week that began w/ vomiting and has caused him to need lots of pain killers & heating pad use. He is thankfully doing much better today. My mom had a breast biopsy, which we will have results on next week. Tuesday she sees an oncologist; they are still investigating the enlarged lymph nodes. I made it through my chemo on Friday w/ flying colors. This is a new protocol. Next Friday & Saturday I return for more chemo. So far I have received one of the two chemos, this Friday they add in the second one. It's called gem/tax for short. Thanks that Chris is feeling better, thanks that all reports on my mom have been positive, thanks that I made it through the chemo! And thanks for your continued prayers.

Love and God bless,
the Alimentis

March 6, 2009

We finally made it out of the clinic and got home only minutes ago. It was a long day (starting @ 9:30 and ending only moments ago). Part of the long day was due to the clinic being backed up as a result of the snow days earlier in the week. We had to wait for the drawn blood results, in queue for the Dr., before we could be seen and then wait for an open space for infusion. The initial attempt at administering Taxotere didn't go well. Carol felt similar pain to what she felt with the Doxil. They backed off the drug and got her comfortable. They gave her some drugs to help minimize the pain and they were able to eventually get the whole bag of Taxotere into her. Then the Gemcitabine was given and it went in well, with minimal burning. They had a warm towel on her arm where the port was installed to help the veins. She is obviously wiped out now and in bed working through the chemo effects. We go back in tomorrow morning for a shot to boost her immune counts. Thanks for your prayers and support. We felt supported throughout the day and were able to move through the events rather peacefully (outside of that initial pain issue, but even then we felt covered). God bless you all, too.

The Alimenti family

March 7, 2009

I am feeling pretty good today, just tired and flushed from all the steroids. I have not experienced any nausea or vomiting. Thank you God. Chris asked us to get him into the clinic on Wednesday a.m. to have his liver checked. We now refer to him as Dr. Alimenti, and yes, he was right on the money. His alt, liver enzyme was 400 above the "suspend all chemo" number. So until his counts recover he is off chemo and feeling better each day. He heads back to clinic on Monday for recheck. On Tuesday, Darcy and I took my mom to an oncologist to follow up on all her scans, ultrasounds, biopsies, and blood work. Additional praises are in order. Mom does not have a metastasized cancer (she has had bladder & colon cancer in the past), nor does she have breast cancer. The kidney bleed is unrelated, but due to papillary necrosis from the use of analgesics, like Aspirin, arthritis pain meds, etc. It should heal in time as she is off those drugs. They did perform blood work as they suspect chronic lymphatic leukemia. We will have results in two weeks. If negative, they will perform a day surgery and remove a lymph node to properly diagnose Low Grade Lymphoma. Although as Chris quipped, "What's the good news in that?" We feel so blessed as both of the above require routine six-month blood checks, no chemo. They basically just watch to ensure her blood counts stay in a healthy range and watch her for infections. So at 82 she is hanging in there and we all feel so blessed to have her in our lives. Darcy keeps teasing her that she has to stay strong as she plans on having her be the flower girl at her wedding. And No, Darcy at this time does not have a perspective beau but we are assured that Our God is working on all those details!! So I am off to the hospital to get my white count boosted up. Thanks for loving on us, thanks for your prayers and thank you, God, for this spring-filled weekend. I took it as my own personal sign from God that He holds us in the palm of His hands. May we all remain in His Hands. God is good and He is a promise keeper.

Love and God Bless,
Carol and family

March 10, 2009

Well, Carol is working through the last treatment and the neutropenic (sp?) shot. Somewhat difficult with the bone pain, a low-grade fever, headache, and it looks like there is some venal redness and soreness where the chemo was injected. But she started feeling better last night and more so this morning. Still a little weak, slight headache, and they'll probably have to use a different vein next time. Chris is doing better, his latest blood sample showed improvement but not enough to put him back on chemo (a double edged blessing). Anyway, he is looking better, starting to eat again and feeling generally stronger. Darcy is working hard with schoolwork, volunteer activities, and play practice, and with everything else she is involved in, she has an SAT test this Saturday so pray for her to do well on that and her SOLs. Thanks again for all your prayers and support, those thoughts and prayers provide the "wind beneath our wings" that helps us soar through this. It's comforting to find peace amid turmoil.

God bless,
The Alimentis

March 10, 2009

I guess I need to emphasize that the "working through" might be an understatement. So you know, the pain is very high in the 1-to-10 scale, and her joints and arm are extremely uncomfortable. Keep praying.

Carol, Tony, Chris, and Darcy

March 12, 2009

Thank you for all the prayers. Today I felt as if I crawled out from under a rock!! I actually felt human again. We saw my doctors and they are going to schedule to have a port inserted as the infusion caused venal irritation. They are also going to do a series of eleven shots vs. the one to boost my white blood count. They feel that the single shot is very strong and is what caused the fever and bone pain. Chris is scheduled to get his blood checked again, 3rd time this week, to see if his liver enzymes are where they should be so he can restart his chemo. They have now vowed to keep both his Methotrexate and 6MP at seventy-five percent and never take it to 100 percent!! Thank you all for your prayers, cards, food, goodies, visits, and love and support. When we can only see the negative, it is your prayers, love, and kindness that make us see the light and remember that God is good, God loves us, and all things are possible through Him.

Love and God bless,
the Alimentis

March 24, 2009

Carol got her port in on Friday and one chemo, she's doing fine right now, Chris is doing well after his monthly Monday treatment. Carol goes in this Friday for the double chemo and will start the multi day white blood cell boost (a variation from the single shot she got a few weeks ago that was too painful). Hopefully this new delivery method will work and the port appears to help in preventing the vein irritation. Carol's mom does have CLL and we are praying for the nonaggressive form. Thanks for your continued prayers.

Carol, Tony, Chris, and Darcy

April 4, 2009

Carol got her double dose of chemo last Friday. She had a few days of discomfort but is on the mend. The Neupogen shots are also going well. We are so thankful. This Friday marks the completion of two cycles of this treatment. Friday, the 10th, she will be scanned to see the effectiveness of the treatments. Our prayers are that this protocol has been effective and they can proceed with the desired six cycles total. We pray for full shrinkage of all the tumors! Chris had an infected toe. He is on antibiotics and is doing much better. Carol's mom, Ann, is having lots of rashes and infections due to her suppressed immune system. Prayers for Chris's and Ann's immune systems to grow stronger. Thank you for all your prayers and support.

Love and blessings,
The Alimentis

April 10, 2009

Thanks for all your prayers and support. We had a long day @ the hospital today. Carol got a couple of CT scans, which showed some significant shrinkage of the large liver tumor. They are watching some new things they found in the scans on the liver, bone, and lungs. She will have more CT scans in seven weeks and they will be scheduling a bone scan. It was a bittersweet day, but worth continuing due to the liver tumor shrinkage. We ask for prayer that the new areas of concern will disappear.

Peace to you,
The Alimentis

April 15, 2009

I Love to report good news! My mom has a form of leukemia. The oncologist was suspecting an aggressive form of the chronic leukemia. But yesterday's blood work revealed that she does not have the aggressive type but a very manageable form. She will not need to be seen for four months. Thank you for your prayers.

God Bless,
Carol, Tony, Chris, and Darcy

April 17, 2009

Carol made it through the two chemos today. Her blood counts were a little low, and she will get them checked again on Monday to see if she needs a transfusion. She starts the neutropenic shots tomorrow and is scheduled for a bone scan on Thursday. Chris had his toe infection dealt with today, and is now on pain and antibiotic medicine in addition to his chemo.

The Alimentis

April 22, 2009

I am referring to myself as a SLUG. I did receive two pints of blood yesterday and today I am beginning to feel the effects. I am so thankful. Tomorrow I have to be at the hospital at 7:30 for a bone scan. This will definitively rule out or confirm new bone lesions. Not sure what that says yet about how they will proceed. My doctor did say he was "perplexed" that my largest tumor in the liver shrunk by two centimeters, yet a new mass has appeared in the liver. Chris in the meantime is experiencing fatigue, loss of appetite, and a rising bilirubin count. He will be rechecked in a week and a half but I will call the clinic on Friday if I do not see some improvement. My mom continues to do well and has been such a help. Tomorrow will be her third day this week escorting us to hospital stays. I thank you for your prayers and I pray blessings upon all of you.

Love & God bless,
Carol & family

April 24, 2009

Thankful, thankful, thankful!! My doctor just called with wonderful news. The bone lesions on the latest CAT scans were NOT confirmed on the bone scan! They had been weeded out through prayer. Thank You, Lord. And thank you to all you prayer warriors. God is so good. So I continue with this protocol and prior to my fifth cycle, in four weeks' time, I will be rescanned. Praying for more weeding out of tumors. I feel such a renewed spirit. I have a dear friend, Pat, currently battling the same cancer. Please pray that Pat's tumors in her lungs dissolve. Chris seems less fatigued. Thank You, Lord.

Love and God Bless,
Carol and family

May 6, 2009

Chris's blood counts were all good. They brought his Methotrexate to 100 percent but have decided to keep his 6MP at seventy-five percent. Hopefully this will prove to be the perfect formula. My last treatment went well and my cousins' visit from Long Island was so special. They left early Sunday and that, thankfully, is when my fever and flu-like symptoms kicked in. But now it is Wednesday and I am past all that nastiness. Friday I receive my next double dose, where my friend, Lynn, from NJ will be with me. It is an all-day affair, so we will have lots of time to catch up. So as always there is much to be thankful for; Chris's counts, the timing of my fever, visits from friends & family, and all of you who hold us up in prayer. Happy Mother's Day to all and remember, if you are not a mother, your birth created a mother, so celebration is for all.

Love and God bless,
Carol

May 17, 2009

We have all been doing well. The kids are getting ready for school ending. Chris has a full clinic day tomorrow, Monday. He receives his twenty-fifth spinal tap. My mom and I will accompany him. I have not been part of his clinic visits for quite some time. It will be nice to be there to support him and see all of the staff. Chris and I go to separate clinics at UVA. My next big day is Friday, the 22nd. I will be scanned, the doctors will review the scans and hopefully they will reveal shrinkages of tumors. Then I will proceed with round five of chemo. Love and God bless to all.

Carol and family

May 22, 2009

Today was a long day between scans & infusions. Carol's scans showed stabilization, which is good. No tumor growth—but no shrinkage. Round five of chemo also started today. The scans did reveal fluid around her lungs, which they feel is a reaction to the chemo. Chris had an ingrown toenail removed so he is limping around. So all in all things are good—God is good and the weather is beautiful! Thanks for your prayers. Please pray that Carol's next scans show tumor shrinkage!!!

Love and God bless,
Tony and gang

May 28, 2009

My chemo has been postponed due to an accumulation of side effects. I am also experiencing pain in my sternum and corresponding back area. Past scans did not show anything so they have scheduled an MRI for Monday morning. I have been bedridden since Monday. Rashes, fever, difficulty breathing, and chest & back pain have been very draining. Most of you know Chris graduates from high school this Thursday and we are having a family celebration on Saturday. I missed an awards ceremony on Tuesday for Darcy. She received five awards for academic excellence. I also missed their play performance. I am feeling so saddened about missing these special events in their lives. Please pray I can be at his graduation. Thank you and God bless.

Love,
Carol

May 28, 2009

Carol has been down—please pray for her. There was some confusion in her message. Chris graduates next Thursday (June 4th) and his celebration follows on Saturday June 6th. Lots of hugs and laughs and thanks for all your notes and prayers.

The "family"

June 2, 2009

My MRI of my spine showed, thank God, NO compression. All my side effects, except for sternum pain, are gone. So thankfully I am feeling much better. And the sternum pain is less today. So I am in good shape for the graduation festivities. I spoke w/my oncologist this a.m. and he does want me to have an X-ray of my sternum & chest tomorrow. But no dye!! He just wants to make sure it's all okay before I get my last dose of round five next week. Thanks for all your prayers and God bless.

Love,
Carol

June 8, 2009

Thank you again for all your prayers. Chris's graduation ceremony & party were wonderful. It was such a nice time to come together and rejoice. We are so proud of him. Due to all the side effects I have experienced, my doctor and I have decided to stop the chemo until sometime in late July/early August. Hallelujah!! I made it through four and a half rounds. They were hoping for six rounds but the disease right now is stable and I was very toxic. So this Friday marks 3 weeks since my last infusion and I should begin to feel better with each passing day. I am going to physical therapy today to try to speed up the recovery. Essentially I have become a SLUG, my legs are like logs and I'm pretty pathetic at getting around. We are in the midst of planning a family vacation to France so I had better get the old bod moving! Our love to all and God bless.

The Alimentis

June 25, 2009

The countdown is on—five days till our French vacation. I had a PET scan this week—only new finding was a small lymph node in neck—will deal w/when I return. More fluid on my lungs so tomorrow I go in for a day procedure to have it drained. Chris's, as we suspected, liver enzymes were highly elevated. No chemo for now, blood work to pinpoint cause and before we leave they will decide if he will be off chemo for the entire trip. Bon voyage!

Amour,
the Alimentis

June 29, 2009

Chris's liver enzymes improved. He has started back on his chemo but at fifty percent. Both our doctors have given us the green light. Thank you for your prayers and au revoir.

Amour,
Carol, Tony, Chris, and Darcy

July 17, 2009

Our vacation was PERFECT! We all had an opportunity to relax and put our cancer issues behind us. We traveled through a countryside that was visually like a storybook. We met folks who opened their hearts to us. Darcy's host family became our family. We felt such warmth. We slept w/our windows open. No humidity and no mosquitoes!!! We toured Monet's garden, which was always on my wish list. We fell in love with "the city of lights." And we have a new appreciation for bread, cheese, and wine. Thank you for all your prayers. We are trying hard to keep that feeling of relaxation but Tony is back on the work treadmill and Chris and I are back at the hospital. Darcy is still in France and we are missing her dearly. Chris is experiencing low platelets, so again chemo has been suspended. He goes back to the hospital on Monday for more testing. I had a new CT scan on Wednesday and will receive the results on Monday. But somehow the change in atmosphere was the medicine we needed to help us move forward in a more peaceful state. We are so thankful we had this opportunity. Again thank you for your prayers, love and support.

God Bless,
the Alimentis

July 24, 2009

Lots of PRAISE reports! Chris and I both had good hospital visits on Monday. Chris's counts were good and he is back on his meds @ fifty percent and doing well. All my tumors are stable—no new metastases and none have grown. So I will be rescanned on two-month intervals and as long as things stay stable, I will not need treatments. I do have increased fluid on both lungs so I am taking an increased dose of diuretics. I feel great and am trying to walk each day. Thanks for the prayers and support.

Carol, Tony, Chris, and Darcy

August 6, 2009

More praises—my lungs have drained!! I need to stay on the diuretics but at half dose. My next scan will be September 9 with doctor visit on the 11th. I am loving this respite. Chris has a big clinic day on August 10th, includes a spinal. But he is doing fantastic, meds still at fifty percent. Thanks for all your prayers.

Love,
Carol, Tony, Chris, & Darcy

August 31, 2009

Today I met with Intervention Radiology to discuss my liver tumor. They presented two options, chemoembolization and an embolization treatment that uses radioactive beads to shrink the tumor. It is nothing we have to act upon ASAP. We have asked that they set up a consult w/a liver surgeon to first rule out resection of the liver tumor, as that has the best prognosis. We have also decided if we did proceed w/some form of embolization we would get a second opinion from Sloan first. So all that said, on the 9th I am scanned, so if you could pray for shrinkage or better yet absence of all tumors that would make the above a moot point. And I will be shouting Amen!!! So on 9/9 please send up prayers for a scan that will show no signs of disease. I feel great, I'm getting hair back, quite grey, and I have lots of energy. It is really hard to believe that I even have cancer. As I tell God every day, "I'm having fun here, can I please stay here a little bit longer." Today I felt He said, "Okay my child." My boy Chris had his Methotrexate tonight. Due to Labor Day his next clinic visit will be on Friday, not Monday. And they will, over the next few weeks, tweak his chemo schedule so that his Methotrexate will be on Thursday nights and his clinic visits will be on Fridays. This schedule will work best with school and work. Chris started at the community college last week and is still at Carmike movie theater. He is so far enjoying school. He is also donning a new coif. He got his hair all chopped off for Locks of Love and is looking quite dapper. Thanks so much for all your prayers and remember me on 9/9.

Love,
Carol, Tony, Chris, and Darcy

September 8, 2009

Boldly and with the encouragement of a friend, and knowing that God is good and God is in control and God loves us, I am asking for prayer for an unbelievable scan tomorrow. A scan that shows my disease shrinking away. Tomorrow is 09-09-09, as some of you have noted. My appointment was scheduled for 10 a.m. I received a call today they want me to arrive at 9 a.m. I know that God's hand is in the midst of all of this and I feel there cannot be a coincidence with all these nines lining up. Someone at church told me when I said the date, 09-09-09, he heard, "benign, benign, benign." Please pray for a miracle. I will have my results on Friday and I will post the outcome. Thank you and God bless.

Love,
Carol

September 11, 2009

Thank You, Lord, for a good report today. The disease is still present but it remains stable. No new metastases and no growth. Hallelujah!! I will be seen monthly for exam & blood work but my CT scans will be on longer intervals, three to four months as opposed to six to seven weeks apart. I am feeling great and so thankful for a God who hears our prayers, never abandons us, and unites our hearts as his army storms the heavens with prayers. So many of you have being praying for me and I am so very grateful for each and every one of you. May you have a wonderfully joyful day.

God Bless, Love,
Carol, Tony, Chris, and Darcy

September 30, 2009

Chris and I are both feeling wonderful. Friday he has a clinic day, no spinal tap this time but lots of chemos. My family was recently all united for my nephew's wedding, which was so special, and everyone could not get over how great Chris looks. And I now have some hair!! Amen and how sweet of God to give me hair that is much nicer than what I had prior to chemo. I did visit w/the liver surgeon recently, a really nice man. Unfortunately, I am not a candidate for surgery because the disease has metastasized too far. The news was bittersweet. On the proddings of my dear friend Pam, I am sending out this info for continued prayer and some specifics regarding my disease. First that God would shrink the tumor in my liver, kidney, and the two spots on my spine. Secondly that God would erase the "shadowings" that they see in my neck lymph node, two lung nodules, pelvic & femur bones, and a secondary liver spot. It sounds like a lot but all things are possible for our ultimate healer. I feel like we, Darcy, Tony, Chris and I, are experiencing a wonderful "grace" period and I am so thankful to all of you for being such faithful servants and bringing our needs to our Lord. God bless you all.

Love,
Carol, Tony, Chris, and Darcy

October 1, 2009

Check out the link below. Our Darcy was interviewed by our local TV channel. Way to go Darcy!!!!! http://www.newsplex.com/video?clipI D=4177859&autoStart=true&contentID=63174342

October 3, 2009

Darcy is the team leader and Chris is the honoree patient for this year's Light the Night Walk for the Leukemia & Lymphoma Society. The walk will take place on Wednesday October 28th starting @ 6 p.m. from the Charlottesville Pavilion. If you would like to donate to leukemia and lymphoma research, you can do that through the link below: http://pages.lightthenight.org/va/Charlva09/darcyalimenti.

Thank you and God bless,
the Alimentis

December 10, 2009

This morning I received a call from my doctor regarding my latest scan and I am so thankful for your love, support, & prayers. All my tumors are stable and one nodule in the lung has shrunk!! I do not have to be scanned again for six months!! This is a true blessing, a gift from God. Yesterday as I laid on the table and received the injection that burnt my veins due to the number of scans I have received this past year, I began to weep silently to God and tell Him how I wanted this to not be a constant part of my life. I prayed for God to remove this cancer, I prayed that this cancer would become an experience I lived through. I thank God for these results and the renewed hope He has given me. Chris also received great news—on March 17th, 2010, his chemo treatments will end!! God is good. May your holidays be blessed with His fruits of love, peace, joy and happiness!

Love,
the Alimentis

December 10, 2009

I forgot to send you all this link on a short film Chris was recently in for the VA Film Fest. Enjoy! http://www.youtube.com/watch?v=EfNfyzHSXgE.

Love,
Carol

March 8, 2010

I have been extremely lax in updating our site. Truthfully things have been going really well. I feel that I should let you know that and not just write when we are in the midst of a major battle. Chris has finished, a little bit earlier than anticipated, his chemo. Thank You, God!! He will be seen in two weeks for a blood check and then things should move to a four-week visit for blood check & pulmonary therapy. The pulmonary stuff will last for six months & the four-week visits stretch to eight weeks after a year. His doctor feels that it will take a good six months for him to really feel what life is like without chemo running through your veins. He is working hard at school & will be in the upcoming play at PVCC. It's a musical, *Clue*. He plays an elderly English housekeeper and even sings a solo. Should be really funny. I am experiencing a period of grace. Doing all my health food stuff and trying to get to the gym several times a week. I can easily slip into a sloth mode, so pray I can keep up the routine. This weekend we went to the memorial service of the only person I knew w/my cancer.

Pat's service was beautiful and I only wish I had had more time to get to know her. Spring is only days away and most of us have experienced a rougher than usual snowfall. So many are welcoming spring with open arms, myself included.

Love and blessings to all,
Carol & family

April 15, 2010

Since I last wrote Chris has been on stage @ PVCC performing as Mrs. White in a musical version of the board game CLUE. He is quite funny playing an elderly English housekeeper. A bit of "Mrs. Doubtfire" with Chris's unique stamp. His last performances are this weekend on Friday & Saturday. Darcy is officially going to attend UVA Nursing School next year. She just received notification that she will be honored by United Way for her volunteer efforts. Thank you Ms. Patty M***** for nominating Darcy. In addition, she received a Super Sibs National Scholarship. So lots of hoorays for Ms. Darcy. Now on to my real need, PRAYER! Chris was sent by oncology to GI doctors due to elevated liver enzymes. Being totally off chemo, it was a perplexing situation to the oncology team. Last week's blood tests ruled out lots of stuff. So thank you Jesus!! Next week, on Wednesday, he will have an ultrasound to RULE OUT A MASS OR NODULE. Please storm the heavens with prayers that the ultrasound comes back normal. Please pray for **NO EVIDENCE OF A MASS OF ANY KIND & NORMAL LIVER COUNTS! AMEN**

God Bless,
the Alimentis

April 23, 2010

Amen!!! The ultrasound was NORMAL!!! They are planning to recheck Chris's labs in two weeks and are expecting to see his liver enzymes return to NORMAL!!! How we love that word—NORMAL. Thank you God and thanks for all the prayers. Have a wonderful weekend.

God Bless,
the Alimentis

September 1, 2010

I know I have not written an entry since April. Yes, **Chris completed his therapy and I have not had any treatments, thank God, since June of '09!!!!** We went to Ireland this June after Darcy's graduation. She went out w/a bang, receiving all kinds of accolades. Ireland was "magical." Unlike in France, I had hair, I did not need those stylish support stockings, and Chris and I hiked with the best of them!! It was a wonderful family vacation that we all hold in our hearts w/sweet memories. Chris has had very low platelet counts, which after six months doctors would have expected to rise into the normal realm, but they have not. So last Friday they performed a bone marrow test to check to see if the leukemia was still active. And again thanking God for His merciful heart, his marrow was great!! Still praying the platelets come up and the issue is that Chris's body takes a little longer than average. My situation has literally grown, the liver and kidney tumors have both grown significantly. My lung nodules have experienced minimal growth but remain there. My spine appears stable. I do have a growth on my tongue, not an unlikely site for this cancer. And I have some spots on both arms. UVA is glad that Tony and I are headed up to Memorial Sloan-Kettering, NYC on Monday. They have scheduled two appointments on the 7th. I will be seeing the head of the sarcoma dept. and a head surgeon to address the tongue growth. Most importantly, we will get their take on what could be done next. We have lots of questions for the NY folks and are unsure how long we will be there. We would love to make a visit to Monmouth County on our way back to VA to see friends and family based on time constraints. It was such a wonderful reprieve from being "sick" this last year. God answered my prayers. When I was first diagnosed I had a son still undergoing chemotherapy and a daughter in high school. Well Darcy is a first year at UVA Nursing School and Chris has completed his course of treatment. In addition, Chris took a filmmaking course at NY Film Academy this summer. He had a blast. He continues this fall at the community college. So I have my children within a five-minute drive of our home. Tony is still gainfully employed. So we have lots to be so thankful for, including wonderful family and friends. I hope you understand my period of silence and I ask for prayer for Tony and I, that we will easily take in what options are available and be guided by the Holy Spirit as to what we should do. Thank you for your prayers. May God be ever present in your lives.

Love,
Carol and family

September 7, 2010

Exhausting day!! We met with the doctors at Memorial Sloan-Kettering. They recommend I start on chemotherapy. The disease has gotten aggressive and needs to be dealt with using systemic treatment. I can have my treatments in VA. They also took off my tongue lesion and will have biopsy results by Friday. The spots on my skin did not look like a problem but they do want me to follow up with a dermatologist. We had a long, but good travel/no glitches. We met wonderful people in NY who are adding us to their prayer list. Tony's best man, Kevin came in last night to have dinner with us. Right now we are in Little Silver w/our dear friends the Salimandos. Tomorrow I hope to see my friend Nancy as well as lots of other Little Silver buddies. Then we will travel twenty minutes south to my brother's and be with them & my mom for a few days. Hoping to connect w/my north Jersey friend, Maryann, as well. So lots of good times to be had. Thank you for your prayers and I will look forward to seeing all you southerners on our return. We felt your prayers and we felt a true sense of peace with all the medical staff. I am ready for the next battle. From Joshua, "Be strong and courageous. Do not be discouraged. Do not be terrified. The Lord will be with you every step of the way." The Lord gave me this scripture just before I left and I have repeated it over and over again. May you all have a great week and when I have more news I'll get back to you.

Love and God bless,
Carol and family

September 10, 2010

Good News! My tongue biopsy came back and it was benign!! We are so thankful. Our trip north has been filled with lots of time spent with family and friends. It has been wonderful to see so many folks we left behind when we moved to Virginia. We need to come up again soon so we can go back to our old church, out to the Island to visit cousins, and Cheri somehow I will connect with you soon! Tomorrow we head back to Charlottesville. Not sure when my treatments will start but I am so thankful for this fun holiday! God is so good. May we all rest in His loving mercies.

Love,
Carol & family

September 16, 2010

No news yet as to when I start the next phase. My doctor is on vacation, so I am enjoying fully this respite!!! Yesterday Tony rented an antique sports car and we journeyed the Blue Ridge Mountains. The owners of this red Alpha Romeo graciously insisted that it be their gift to us, as they have survived seventeen years and counting a cancer diagnosis!! The day was peaceful. We seemed to have the road to ourselves, and the weather was picture perfect. Thanks again to the generous hearts of others. Life is GOOD! Thanking God for all the blessings He has bestowed upon us! May you feel His presence today.

Love and God bless,
Carol

September 19, 2010

Tony and I attended a wonderful one-day retreat in DC for cancer survivors. There was sharing our stories, info on nutrition, stress reduction, yoga, and art therapy and so much more. We left with a renewed hope. We also, with much prayer, have decided to not start any treatments until next week. We want this week to be a time of celebration, as Chris turns twenty on Tuesday. It is so weird to think of him as no longer a teenager! We will fetch Darcy from school and have a family dinner this coming weekend. We also want to talk with the doctors this week about a different approach to my treatments. We feel more comfortable with surgically removing the kidney tumor, which can be done laparoscopically. Next the surgical removal of the liver tumor. This will be a bigger ordeal but I am feeling quite strong at this time. After the surgeries, then begin some chemotherapy. We will meet with doctors this week and discuss this approach. We ask for prayer and peace as we walk through this next phase.

Love and God bless,
Carol & family

September 22, 2010

Ah the world of oncology! Today did not go exactly as I foresaw but dialogue has opened. The oncology perspective is that the risks associated with surgical procedures does not outweigh any possible benefits due to the level of my disease. But I am being sent for 3 consults, one w/an oncology dermatologist to look at my arm growth, one w/the kidney surgeons to again discuss removal of the kidney tumor, and finally back to the liver surgeons. My doctor will also bring my case before the tumor board. After much discussion our doctor is somewhat comfortable w/the kidney resection as that is a laparoscopic procedure and could offer more data to the mix. He is going to try to get all this in motion and have us meet back with him in a two- to three-week timeframe. We also discussed chemotherapy options and he had some openness to trying some less conventional options. We are praying and we ask for prayer, that Our Lord, the Great Physician, will direct my course of treatments. So another respite from treatments, hooray!!!

Love you all and God bless,
Carol & family

October 8, 2010

On the Alimenti health front, Chris is looking great!! Skinny, beyond skinny, and platelets still low, in fact, new level was 85. So still need prayers that they do a miraculous rebound, 150 to 450 is normal range. Chris had a rash on his neck. Got on the Internet and our investigations led us to the diagnosis, Shingles! Diagnosis confirmed yesterday. Started on treatment. The good news, it has been caught early. Next, a TB outbreak out at his college, so he is getting tested for that today!!! My doctors have either abandoned me because I was a misbehaving patient or the oncology wheels are churning slowly. Whatever the reason, I am allowing for the reprieve and telling my body to heal. Someone told me to think of myself as a cat and just lie around all day. So I am a self-proclaimed SLUG. Not a bad way to get out of household chores. We have also decided not to do chemo, or at least the options that have been presented thus far. My cancer, ULMS, does not respond well and neither did I to the drugs. The percentages are less than thirty percent chance of shrinkage, of which I saw NADA on my first two attempts. And sadder yet is reoccurrence happens on average eight to twelve months post treatment. So I am in the complimentary therapy realm; vegetarian, restfulness, enemas, and lots of meditation time. Much more doable and with this time off, we can measure its effectiveness. Nothing to lose! Enjoying this glorious autumn weather. May every rustle of the leaves bring you closer to Our Creator.

Love and God Bless,
Carol and family

November 7, 2010

Lots of activity in the Alimenti household. Chris is over the bout w/ shingles. Amen! His platelets are still low 90s but because his marrow & all his other blood work is fine they just think that Chris, as a result of treatment, might have a new low, but not to be confused w/ dangerous. So that also is an answer to prayer. Chris just completed a seventy-two-hour VA Adrenaline Film Festival Project. What an ordeal. He and his team did great. They rec'd a mentor award and were third in the jury choice. Best of all they had a blast. Soon I will have a web site where you can view their creation. I have been up & down but as of lately encouragement is reigning thank You, Lord. We experienced a wonderful UVA parent weekend w/ Darcy. They had a pinning ceremony for first-year nursing students, breakfast at the pavilion, personally met the new president, spent time meeting her friends, just a glorious weekend. Another answer to prayer, she is so happy at school! Tony and I will head to Illinois on December 1 & 2 for a consult at the Block Center for Integrative Cancer Treatment. I have lots more doctor visits and paperwork to gather till then. Liver surgeon, dermatologic oncologist, and most importantly, a November 22nd CAT scan, praying that all those buggers would disappear! But all in all I have very little discomfort, just fatigue and fighting off the negative voices that try to chase me down rabbit holes. But I am thankful for all who share in our journey and I pray that you will all experience His love and peace and may it penetrate your hearts. I'll post my scan results sometime after the 22nd.

Blessings,
the Alimentis

November 23, 2010

I just reread the surgical report of September 2009. At that time surgery was ruled out, evidence of metastasized disease included traces on the liver, kidney, lungs, spine, pelvic, femur, and neck lymph node. I have received no traditional treatments since June 2009. Monday's scan shows disease in the kidney & liver ONLY! I am now a surgical candidate. This is a big deal. My cancer does not respond to chemo well and neither did I. My best odds of gaining some time here w/a good quality of life are through surgical removal w/clear margins. It is not considered a cure but it has always been my best option, if possible. So God has opened this door and miraculously vanished tumors. Thank you for standing with us in prayer and for your words of encouragement. I still have some hurdles to go through but God willing, surgery should happen prior to Christmas. Both sites will be done in tandem and it will require approx. One week hospital stay and three to four weeks recovery time. I will then be carefully monitored. On a very somber note, but with strong faith that God is good and merciful, yesterday we took my mom to the hospital. She is 84, she has CLL, chronic leukemia, she has suffered multiple strokes, and has survived bladder and colon cancers, to name just a few of her past medical traumas. She is, as many of you can testify, a pillar of strength with a heart that is rich and full of love. She is currently in ICU and is "a very sick person." She is septic, working on getting her blood pressure up and receiving transfusions. The medical team tells us things could very easily take a turn for the worse. It has been a grueling two days but we saw the tenacious spirit still reigning in her this evening. We are not sure, as in all life situations, how things will turn out, but our prayer is that God is tender and merciful to our mother, whom we so dearly love. Please keep her in your prayers.

Happy Thanksgiving to all and God bless,
the Alimentis

November 30, 2010

My mom spent four touch & go days in ICU, four additional days in the hospital, and today was taken by ambulance to rehab! It was not her time, although she was ready, God has other plans. Please pray that our mother will grow stronger each day, especially her compromised breathing and that when the Lord does come for her, it will be a peaceful passing. Today, after visiting with three doctor offices, I know for certain that God is very active in the healing arena. Several of the medical staff expressed awe that I am still here and that I am now a surgical candidate. Thank You, Lord, for allowing me more time here to watch my children grow and evolve. Things in the medical world are not always as simple as I would naively assume. Our livers are lopsided. The bad part of mine is in the large side and the puny side is the good one. My good one is just too puny to jump into surgery, only twenty percent would be left. So on Monday I will be hospitalized for only one night to have a procedure called Portal Vein Embolization. It will take two to four hours, they will close off the portal vein blood supply to bad side of liver. Good side is fooled and thinks it needs to start growing; they are hoping for a doubling in size. Four to five weeks later they come back and scan and God willing, the bad liver side, along w/the gall bladder, can finally get cut out. The Portal Vein Embolization will cause a week's worth of vomiting & flu-like symptoms. Please pray that I can handle the procedure and the side effects from it. The kidney tumor waits till complete recovery occurs and then it gets the axe. So more battle wounds in my future but how sweet is God to allow me to have a future. Again they say this is not curative, but the way God has been erasing tumors, only God knows for certain. So my heartfelt thanks for storming the heavens, God is healing and God is good!!!

Love & God Bless,
Carol and family

December 6, 2010

Carol got out of surgery today after ~ four hours getting the PVE. She is doing well, in good spirits and working on getting much needed rest. She is scheduled to be let out of the hospital mid-day tomorrow. Then it is rest and left liver lobe building time! She will be feeling pretty sick for a week or so as the liver is now @ ~ twenty percent and working on growing and filtering. So prayers for healthy liver growth and minimal sickness and lots of rest are greatly appreciated. Last week we had a very productive trip to Chicago and were very pleased with the treatment options and information provided by the doctors. The nutritionist provided a very detailed adjustment to our nutrition and supplement regimen to help good liver growth and prepare Carol's body for fighting the tumors. Thanks again for all your continued support, prayers and well wishing.

Peace and Grace to you all,
Tony & Family

December 7, 2010

A quick update on our mom. She is doing better. She still has a long road ahead. She still has a lot of fluid issues but has been spending time in a chair and doing some exercises in the chair w/physical therapy which, along w/the Lasix, should improve the situation. Her spirits were better today. The doctors goal is to get her back on her feet and to be walking with a cane.

Carol: I am home and I have experienced no pain. In fact, I was hooked up to a pain pump but miraculously did not need to use it. I did need oxygen but they weaned me off it this morning I have also not experienced any of the other nasty side effects they predicted. So again, thank you for your prayers. Heading off for a nap!

Love and God bless,
Carol & family

December 12, 2010

My mom, Ann, will be coming home on Thursday. It has been quite an ordeal; she was hospitalized on November 22nd. She will be in a wheelchair till therapy and her body grows stronger and on oxygen. Please pray that our home renovations will, miraculously, be completed to accommodate a wheelchair. She is growing stronger each day but being home will be the best medicine. Also prayer is needed for the fluid issue to resolve itself. My procedure on Monday went off without a hitch. I spent the night at the hospital and never even needed the pain pump. In addition, I have not had to use the anti-nausea or pain meds they sent me home with. I have some fatigue but that should pass in a week's time. I am scheduled to be scanned on January 3. The surgical date is January 17th based on that scan. Now it's just my left liver lobe. GROW, GROW, GROW! Thank you for your continued prayers and support.

God bless,
Carol and family

December 16, 2010

I had to laugh or I would be in tears. We woke up today to snow and the wheelchair transport was not working due to the weather. We did get her home. Hooray!!! They sent her with oxygen but she has not needed it as of this writing. She is resting comfortably, hospital bed arrived one hour prior to her arrival. The bathroom renovations are almost complete, tile behind the bathtub and fixing the floor. But for now a bedside commode is doing the job just fine. She has a brand spanking new wheelchair; she is not doing wheelies yet! Pray that she can hear again. Her cough and congestion have left her nearly deaf. We are writing everything down and it frustrates her. And prayers that she grows stronger each day. The good news is, I have not been obsessing w/ my situation, no pity parties allowed, and Chris's platelets rose to 105!!! So lots to be thankful for and yes, the snow is beautiful.

Stay warm and God bless,
Carol & family

December 22, 2010

This Christmas is teaching us many lessons in what this season represents. Your prayers for my mom are being answered. Each day she grows stronger. We are so thankful for your love and support. We wish you all a Blessed Christmas, filled with His love, peace and joy! Below is a link to our Christmas ecard.

Love and God bless,
the Alimentis
http://www.americangreetings.com/ecards/view.pd?i=525396923&m=2866&rr=y&source=ag999

January 4, 2011

My mom has been getting stronger each day! No oxygen, no wheelchair. She climbed four steps today and uses the walker like a champ. She still has some edema but even that is getting much better. Thank you for all your prayers. God is so good. I had my scan yesterday but I have not heard back yet as to how things look. I will probably hear tomorrow so if you can send up the prayers for a strong left liver lobe growth I would be so grateful. I did my pre-operation tests today and that also went smoothly. Surgery is scheduled for January 17th. Despite the chill in the air, life feels so good. Happy New Year to all and may you and yours be blessed with a healthy and joyful year.

Love and God bless,
Carol and family

January 6, 2011

Surgery is a go!!! January 17th is the date. I do not have an exact percentage number for the increase yet, but have been told things are good to move forward. Being the control freak that I am, I wanted the exact info. I guess God continues to work on my surrendering, sometimes I feel like a lost cause! Thank you Jesus for prayers answered yet again!! My mom is doing great but unfortunately the two units of blood she received eleven days ago, did not boost her red blood cells enough. In fact, they are still going in the wrong direction. Not sure what the next move will be. Hope to learn more on that subject tomorrow. For now I hold on to a favorite verse, "Don't worry about tomorrow for tomorrow will have enough worries of its own." Thanks for all your prayer and support.

Love,
Carol & family

January 12, 2011

More info on my surgery, still on for the 17th, Monday! My liver in twenty-four days grew from 330 cc's to 912 cc's. So the volume was twenty percent of the total liver and it is now thirty-five percent. It will have had an additional fourteen days to beef up from the latest scan to the surgery, so it will be a great size by the time they lop off the right side. So once again lots of praises to sing out. Thank You, Lord. My mom continues to surprise us with her recovery. She did take a fall yesterday, trying to wrap a large throw around herself while standing, not a good idea. She has a slight sprain in her ankle. Her OT, thankfully, also works at the ski resort for the rescue squad and checked it out today. She will be working more on balance issues now and of course mom will be more cautious. She is even going to have her learn to get herself up after a fall on her own!!! We are praying that will not be necessary. Lots of wintery weather all over the country, so I hope everyone is staying warm. Again thanks for your love and your prayers.

God Bless,
Carol & family

January 17, 2011

So much to be thankful for today! The doctors had decided that they would check around once Carol was open to be sure there were no other tumors to deal with and thankfully there were no new ones found so they proceeded with the surgery. She was finishing up around 4 and now at 6:30 she is in a room. Please pray for continued recovery and relief from pain. Thank you for your prayers!

Love and God Bless,
Darcy

January 18, 2011

Carol is recovering well. They had her sit up today. She's still in a lot of pain, but the meds and sleep are helping. One note on the liver tumor they took out: the doctor said it was about the size of a cantaloupe and had also gotten a little bit into the left side. However, it was still in a good spot (God is looking out for her), and they were able to get it all and not compromise the left side. The hope and prayer is that the remaining liver will grow to a normal liver size. We continue to pray that she will continue to recover, get some much needed restorative sleep, no complications, and minimal soon to end pain. Thanks for your continued support and prayers, may God's blessings be 100 fold back to you for all you've given us.

The Alimentis

January 28, 2011

Carol is continuing on the road to recovery. It's a long road, she is experiencing a lot of fatigue and various aches and pains. However, she was able to move around more these past two days than she did last week. She still needs a lot of rest and prayers. Thanks for all your thoughts, prayers, and support.

God Bless,
The Alimentis

February 8, 2011

I am so thankful for all your prayers, notes, food, love, and support. This was tougher than I could ever have imagined. But I am through the worst for now. I was feeling great despair but now I feel comfort and know that I have not been forsaken. Such little faith. God is good. My mom continues to impress all the therapists with her remarkable progress. She is a great example of persevering. The tumor grew quickly and in order to get clear margins they had to cut into the left lobe a little, while removing the right lobe. But the best news is all clean cells, no additional cancer was found in that area. Thank You, Lord. I will see the doctors next Tuesday and know more about the scheduling of the kidney surgery. But I am reassured to learn that it will not involve any rib manipulations, as the liver did!!

Love and God bless,
Carol and family

February 20, 2011

March Madness! The kidney surgeon called me Friday night and my next surgery is scheduled for March 11th. I figured I might as well just jump in and get it behind me. This March also marks Chris's first anniversary from chemo. His continued low platelet level has his team scheduling a bone marrow test for March 18th. We are just praying that the leukemia has created a new norm for his platelet levels. So prayers are needed that the bone marrow test reveals beautifully clear, healthy marrow! My mom has surpassed all of the medical staff's expectations. She is up and down the stairs and looking great. She has had to resume blood pressure meds and experienced a mini stroke last week. We are praying that all her heart/pressure issues miraculously smooth out and no hospital visits are necessary. We are, as I imagine many of you are, awaiting spring. I plan to plant pansies this week so I will be greeted by their smiling faces after my surgery. I started driving on Friday, so my mom and I have been getting out. So life is good and life is full of challenges. We are thankful for all of you who stand with us as we embrace life's bumps. A friend recently gave me a plaque that reads: ***"Life is not about waiting for the storm to pass. It is about learning to dance in the rain."*** Praying that our hearts, minds, and feet are free to dance.

Love and God bless,
Carol & family

March 8, 2011

Pansies are planted and I even tackled some of those dreaded spring chores like freezer cleaning! I met w/the kidney surgeon yesterday and all is a go for Friday. The surgery is bigger than I thought. Larger incision, longer hospital stay, longer recovery, rib manipulation and two days of clear liquids prior to surgery! Whenever I start to not feel like a sick person, it seems like I am reminded that I have this nasty disease. Please pray that there are no complications, that the doctors get clear margins and that their poking around they find no additional cancer and that I can fight the battle with His rod and staff to comfort me. Enjoy the whispers of spring ascending upon us.

Love and God Bless,
Carol and Family

March 12, 2011

After a long day, Carol made it to a room around 7:30 last night (we entered the admissions room @ 9:45 a.m.). The only hitch was a delay in starting due to a change in anesthesia methodology to be used. Surgery started around 1:30, and they were able to remove the tumor with clear margins!!! Initial testing of the surrounding remaining kidney showed negative for cancer!!! Plus, the partial nephrectomy was possible, leaving more than half the kidney!!! There were no complications during the process, nor in closing her back up!!! They sent the tumor and samples for pathology analysis and we should hear those results around Wednesday. Carol had a great sense of peace and joy last night and expressed a lot of praise and thankfulness for the love, prayers, and blessings from you, and God's will in this process. She's very tired and will be in the rest & recovery phase for a few days. She's on a lot of pain meds right now as they had to cut between and move back some ribs due to the kidney being higher up in her abdomen, possibly pushed up by the tumor which was on the lower end of the kidney. So, thanks for your continued prayers & support. Keep them coming, for her continued recovery. We'll update more when we see how today plays out. Thanks again, God bless & peace to you, too!

The Alimentis

March 18, 2011

One week post surgery and all is well. "His mercies are new every morning," was my chant as I showered for the first time in a week. The day before I felt like a carved up carcass and cried myself to sleep, and I woke renewed. He hears our prayers, He feels our tears, He loves us so much. Thank You, Lord! Today Chris was scheduled for a bone marrow test, but guess what? They decided it wasn't necessary. His platelets were at 94, which is about an average number for the last year but they said he's fine. And he is fine. So another Amen! Spring officially arrives tomorrow, may we all be mesmerized by the way God wakes up the earth in such a show of glory.

Love and God bless,
Carol and family

April 6, 2011

I overdid things and I am now looking at a hernia. ICK! I am being very careful now, with lifting, etc. Things are working in the plumbing area, so no emergency. They will wait till I heal from the surgery before they deal w/the hernia. Praying it will miraculously disappear.

Love and God Bless,
Carol & family

April 23, 2011

May the peace and joy of the Risen Christ be with you at Easter and always.

Love and God Bless,
the Alimentis

April 25, 2011

We just returned from the doctor with good news! I do not have a hernia. I have dropped some weight w/both surgeries and the bulging is just muscle and bowel that is protruding and very obvious due to the weight loss. It will take several months till it is all settled down. In the meantime, I must be very careful and limit my exercise to walking and give the abdominal area a complete rest. Chris is scheduled for a bone marrow test on May 13th. They want to be sure that no relapsing has occurred. He looks great and we are prayerful and thankful in advance, nothing is wrong, Thanks for all the prayers, love and support through the years.

Love and God Bless, Carol and family

May 13, 2011

Thank You, Lord!!!! Today Chris was scheduled for a bone marrow test. As we were driving over to the hospital I said that I think your platelets are going to be @ 120 and they will cancel the test. They were 130!!! They finally made a decent jump closer to normal. Not only was the test cancelled, but he is now on a two-month check-up versus four weeks!!! I continue to recover each day at a remarkable rate. I am walking a lot and have resumed most of my activities. I will have an MRI on 6/13 with a follow-up with my oncologist on the 20th. Prayerfully thankful that my MRI will read NED (No Evidence of Disease)! Although it is raining outside we are feeling God's sunshine reigning in our hearts. Thanks for all your prayers.

Love and God Bless,
Carol & family

June 15, 2011

Monday I had my MRI w/contrast to see what was lurking. Your prayers were felt as I underwent the testing and felt such peace. Even now as I review the radiology report I feel the peace of Christ. On many levels the report was positive. The kidneys, liver, and lungs show no concerns. My pancreas does have multiple lesions. I will learn more on my office visit on the 20th. Pray for wisdom for the doctors regarding how to proceed.

Love and God bless,
Carol & family

June 20, 2011

Saw the oncologist today. He was very pleased with my recent scan, as the kidney and liver looked great. He is, however, forwarding my scan to the oncology surgeon to review the pancreas lesions. It is the same surgeon who operated on my liver. He did say that it is another big surgery, called Whipple, to remove them. But I am hoping that the surgeon will have other options, that are less invasive. Hoping also, because the lesions are small, and they may take a wait and see policy. I will post again after I meet w/the surgeon, but it may be a while as Tony and I are headed to Italy for the first two weeks of July. We are getting excited about our trip. Thanks again for your prayers. God is goooood!!!

Love and God bless,
Carol & family

June 30, 2011

The surgeon feels we can watch & wait. Sounds good to me. Tony & I are off to Italy for some R&R. I did update Sloan-Kettering with what is going on so I can get a sarcoma specialist's take on my scans. Never hurts to get a second opinion. Enjoy the summer.

Love and God bless,
Carol & family

July 19, 2011

Italy was MOLTO BENE! We met our long time friends, the Salimandos, at the Rome airport and headed up to a quaint olive growing region just forty miles north. The scenery was magnificent, the people were genuine, and the food was delectable. (Check out the new Italy photos.) The journey home was long but the kids fared great w/o us, of course! Chris's platelets took another dip into the nineties, so mid-August a bone marrow test is again scheduled. Praying his blood work will rectify itself and the test will not be necessary. I heard from Sloan-Kettering and they do not feel that they have anything more to offer in way of treatment or advice. Basically they shut the door. But I am looking at it as a positive, I get to sit still and let UVA and all my alternative stuff, bathed in prayer, wash over me. I feel great and intend to just enjoy all that the Lord has placed before me: family, friends, and nature. God Bless and stay cool!

Love,
Carol & family

August 10, 2011

Friday morning Chris has a bone marrow test. Please pray that his marrow shows no signs of leukemia!

Thank you and God Bless,
Carol & family

August 11, 2011

Chris's oncologist just called to reschedule his bone marrow test to 8/18, Thursday @ 1:45. She had a new emergency patient, ugh!!! More time to send prayers upward for Chris and her newest patient. Chris is still seen in pediatric oncology, so the new patient is a young one. Thanks to all you prayer warriors.

Love and God bless,
Carol & family

August 16, 2011

I just posted some photos of Chris's car. On Sunday night while he was driving through Charlottesville a micro storm caused a tree to fall on his vehicle while he was in it. He, miraculously, walked away uninjured. We believe that his being kept safe was the result of all the prayers that have been sent up in his name. Our Lord is keeping him in the palm of His hand. We are thankful and humbled by Our Savior's grace.

Love and God bless,
Carol & family

August 20, 2011

NO CANCER!!! We are thankful for all the prayers prayed for Chris. His test results were negative for leukemia of all types. Thank you all for pressing in and believing in God's mercy and healing hand.

Love and God bless,
Carol

August 30, 2011

Another bump in the road. Last Wednesday a.m., Chris ran straight into a parked bus. He lost consciousness and today's visit at neurology confirmed our suspicions, epilepsy. Chris has had a low threshold for seizure activity since birth and the possibility of having full-blown epilepsy was always a threat. He started on his seizure meds today. They wean him onto the meds over a four-week time frame. We are so thankful that no one was seriously injured. The car is totaled and Chris will not be able to drive until he is seizure free for six months. So he will have to put up with his parents chauffeuring him around! Once again Chris has been held in the palm of HIS HAND! Thank you Jesus! Please pray for no adverse side effects to the meds and for Chris to emotionally and mentally process the last few weeks of life's bumps. I head in to see the oncologist on 9/12 for a checkup. Praying that I get a good report.

Love and God bless,
the Alimentis

September 14, 2011

Good News! Chris had an MRI to rule out brain tumors and all was clear. He also seems to be handling the anti-seizure meds without any adverse side effects. Still needs emotional and spiritual uplifting. I saw my oncologist and he moved up my scans from December to Monday due to some abdominal issues. He thinks the huge cavity left behind from the surgeries is now home to a section of my colon and it is somewhat knotted up. But to err on the safe side he wants to do the scanning sooner. Also he thinks the pancreatic lesions are like polyps in your colon, if left alone they become, over time, malignancies. He does not think they are metastasized leiomyosarcoma but budding pancreatic cancer. Neither sounds like an option I would choose and regardless they will be watched. Please continue to lift up Chris and pray for discernment for my doctors and radiologists as they try to figure things out. God is sooooo good. Praying that you all enjoy this upcoming favorite season, autumn!

Love and God bless,
Carol

September 21, 2011

Good News! My CT scan shows no new lesions, a clean liver and kidney and stable spine and pancreas readings. There was some growth of one of the three nodules in my lungs. Not too bad! We are rejoicing! Thanks for your prayers.

Love and God Bless,
Carol & family

December 25, 2011

Wishing you all a Merry Christmas! Thank you for all your prayers, love and support over the years. Chris made it to his five-year marker this November and I made it to the three-year mark the same month!! Much to be thankful for, especially the love of family and friends. May you all enjoy peace, love, and health through our Lord Jesus.

Blessings,
the Alimentis

February 29, 2012

I wanted to send you all a health update. I know it has been a while, which is a good thing, no problems. Here is the update: Chris will have an isotope nuclear test on Thursday. But it looks like Graves and medication can sometimes kick the thyroid into neutral. If not, in three months they will either radiate or surgically remove his thyroid. He is bummed w/yet another health problem. Please pray that the meds will do the trick and for his emotional well-being. On my front, the chest scan is still watching four nodules, the largest is 8mm, which is still tiny, thank You, God! The abdomen MRI shows the pancreas lesions as stable. They did find a new tumor, 1.4 cm (this is still tiny) on the right kidney. To give you a reference point, I had forty percent of the left removed last March, a 4.3 cm tumor. They also found bone infiltration at L1, but still tiny. I have had spinal lesions at T10, 11, & 7 in the past and surgery and radiation has left them disease free. So all in all, it was a good report. Things are small and will be followed. The chest will be rescanned in six months and the abdomen will be MRIed in three months. And continued praises my platelets were 147 and the white blood cells are nearly 6, which is really miraculously up from the past counts. These are all great numbers! So if you can pray that the L1 bone be cleared of cancer and the chest nodules disappear and the right kidney tumor melt away! And the pancreas lesions dissolve! Amen. Thank you all for your prayers, I feel God's hand upon me and I feel tremendous peace.

Love and God bless you all,
Carol and family

June 10, 2012

My mother had turned her final corner and leaped into our Savior's loving arms this past Friday. We all will miss her dearly. She is a very special lady. Her body simply grew weaker and now she can thankfully, rest peacefully. She did not want to be a burden despite our continual assurance that it was our privilege to share our home with her these last years. With Chris getting ready for a twelve-month film program starting July 5th in NYC, Darcy working for the summer at Duke's oncology center and me scheduled for another kidney resection on July 13th, I believe my mom asked God to take her and God in His mercy said yes. "All is well with my soul for my God is in control. I know not His plans but I know my soul is in His hands."

Love and God bless,
Carol and family

July 12, 2012

Chris is officially a New Yorker! He is all settled and busy with his film program. Darcy is enjoying her Duke experience. Tony and I are officially empty nesters. We miss my mom dearly but we are embracing this next phase of life. On the medical front, tomorrow I go for my sixth surgery associated with this cancer not counting the port in and out. But who's counting, right! This one is identical to the last partial nephrectomy, except on the opposite side. Same surgeon, whom I really love. I do have to be opened, due to past surgical adhesions, laparoscopic procedure was not available. So this Friday the 13th please send some prayers up to heaven that all goes well. God has given me lots of peace about the surgery, but not so much about the prep I am about to start drinking—really yucky!!

Love and God Bless,
Carol

July 13, 2012

Thanks for all your thoughts, well wishes, and prayers. Carol made it through the surgery very well. The doctors were very happy with the outcome. Very little bleeding, so a transfusion wasn't needed, while they did find a second (but much smaller) tumor right next to the one they were going after, they got them both. The Dr. said she looked over and felt around the kidney and did an ultrasound to make sure there weren't other tumors hanging around the kidney and didn't find any. Carol is resting comfortably (probably due to the meds as the Dr. wants her to rest a lot, at least two days to let the nerves calm down) actually pretty much sleeping except when the pain kicks in, then she wakes up and presses the "button." It was a long day, checked in @ 10:30 and got to her room about 9. If she gets a lot of rest and recovers well, the Dr. said she should be able to go home sometime Monday. So, thanks again for all your prayers and support. We are blessed by you all. Thank you and peace be with you, too.

Tony

July 15, 2012

I am home!!!! I am somewhat sore but that's what pain meds are for! I plan to take it easy, read some good books and just relax. The only exercise I can do for six weeks is walking. But I think all the workouts I did prior have really made this surgery very do-able. Pathology report should be ready by Wednesday. Thank you all again for your prayers. We have a faithful, loving and awesome GOD!

Carol

July 25, 2012

I am recovering well. My motto has been Healing & Hibernation but I am now beginning to venture back out into the world. My staples were removed on Monday. The pathology report came back. They removed two tumors, both metastasized leiomyosarcoma. Not any big surprise but was glad they looked so carefully and found the second tumor lurking, it was a tiny one, only 0.7 cm. They ultrasounded the kidney while I was open and my doctor said they had six sets of eyes scoping it to make sure they got everything. So all looks clear. Again praise and thanks to Our Lord and Savior for His grace & mercy.

Love and God bless,
Carol

August 15, 2012

Just had an oncology visit and chest scan. All the teeny nodules in lungs are pretty much unchanged. My platelets are still low, 91 but up from my leaving the hospital, at 82. My liver enzymes are very slightly elevated. All things they will watch. In this chest scan they can also see the upper part of my spine. The old sites of metastasis where I had surgery & radiation are thankfully stable. There is a new spot of concern—"cortical erosion of the posterior wall of T8 vertebral body." They will rescan in two months, if things are worse my doctor recommends radiation, which I had on other spinal lesions and it did the trick. He also talked about an oral chemo, taken daily, called Pazopanib, which has shown some promise in slowing down the disease progression. So I have some homework researching this new drug option. On the kid front, Darcy is home from Duke. She had a great summer experience and is gearing up for UVA fall semester. Chris is in full throttle in NYC working on his film studies. Tony and I spend our time visiting our children and enjoying this phase of parenting. Praying you are all healthy and happy.

God Bless,
Carol & family

October 23, 2012

I am scheduled for yet another surgery. Sounds crazy. My oncologist says I am keeping the surgeons in business! Not my plan. My latest site of activity is back in the spine. It is the area in the thoracic above where they removed the tumor nearly four years ago. T7 & T8 are being targeted. The area had been radiated four years ago, which makes reradiating not a great option. So on November 7th I will have a surgery which will remove those two vertebrae and replace them with an expandable cage, sixteen screws, and two rods. They say this is a big one, bigger than any past surgeries. I humbly request your prayers. Prayers for no complications, surgeons' hands guided by Our Lord, and a speedy recovery. Thank you for walking with us all these years. We feel truly blessed.

Love and God bless,
Carol & family

November 8, 2012

Today is a day to be thankful. My mom had her surgery—six hours later she has two less vertebrae, the cancerous tumors were removed, and the sixteen screws and pins, the rod from T4-T12, and the expandable cage are now in place. She is still in the ICU, but she can move all her limbs. She has had eight blood transfusions, two bags of platelets, and two bags of plasma. She will hopefully be moved to the floor unit tomorrow. Everyone is amazed at how wonderful she is doing. God is good! So, thank you all for your prayers and support. Please continue to pray for her and her recovery: that her strength will be renewed, her pain will be minimal, her spirit will remain positive, and that she will continue to be filled with the peace of the Holy Spirit. Thank you everyone for your continued support over the years.

Love and God Bless,
Darcy

November 15, 2012

Carol had to go back in the hospital overnight. She had an ileus, which is a bowel obstruction. They were able to clear things up and she was discharged today. She has slept all day as she is exhausted. Now it is rest and recuperation time. Thanks again for your prayers.

Love,
Tony & family

November 20, 2012

My Mom has had a bit of a bumpy recovery. After she was discharged on the 13th she was readmitted on the 14th, then discharged again on the 15th and then spent all of the 16th in the emergency room. All of the complications were related to the surgery. She is currently at home and the last few days have been going well. She finally seems to be on the road to recovery. We are very thankful this Thanksgiving for all of your prayers and support and her continued healing.
Love,
Darcy
P.S. Have a Wonderful Thanksgiving.

December 24, 2012

Merry Christmas from our house to yours, wishing you a season of light, love, hope, and peace.

Love and God Bless Carol,
Tony, Chris, Darcy, and Oscar
"Peace to you and your house! Peace to all that is yours!" 1 Sam. 25:6

January 16, 2013

As you know Darcy is in her third year at the UVA nursing school. She is very passionate about her career journey. She wants to work in the oncology area. Last summer she did an externship at Duke's gynecology/oncology clinic. She wants to truly understand her patients so she can be a compassionate caregiver. She has decided to participate in the cause she describes below. Please do not feel any pressure to participate but do pray that God's hand is fully involved in this and all of her nursing choices.

Love and God bless,
Carol

Dear Friends and Family,

As you know, many of my loved ones and dear friends have battled cancer. This March I'm having my head shaved to stand in solidarity with kids fighting cancer, but more importantly, to raise money to find cures. Please support me with a donation to the St. Baldrick's Foundation. This volunteer-driven charity funds more in childhood cancer research grants than any organization except the U.S. government. Your gift will give hope to infants, children, teens, and young adults fighting childhood cancers. So when I ask for your support, I'm really asking you to support these kids. Thank you! Click "Make a donation" to give online, or donate by phone or mail. http://www.stbaldricks.org/participants/alimenti4cure.

Thank you for your support,
Darcy Alimenti
"Some days there won't be a song."

February 10, 2013

Dear Friends, Family, and Loved Ones,

Tomorrow my mom is going to have a CT scan and then will be meeting with her oncologist to discuss the findings. Please pray that her scan will show no disease progression. Please pray that there will be no new tumors. Please pray that the tumors will be stable or decreased in size. Thank you for all your support, prayers, and love.

Love and God Bless,
Darcy

> *"And God shall wipe away all tears from their eyes; and there shall be no more death, neither sorrow, nor crying, neither shall there be any more pain: for the former things are passed away." Revelation 21:4*

February 11, 2013

Carol met with the Doctors today and the pain in her hip is due to the tumor breaking through the bone and into the soft tissue. We will consult with radiology to discuss the next step. There has been a sensitive spot on her scalp that is now a raised area. They are setting up a consult with a dermatologist to have it surgically removed as they believe it to be a metastasis. Tumors in the lungs and other organs look stable. Please pray that these two above procedures can be successfully executed and minimally invasive. Thank you for your prayers.

Tony and family

February 18, 2013

Tomorrow we head to UVA for scans, markings, and round one of radiation. As it turned out they found two bone metastases on my left hip that have grown out of the bone into the soft tissue. They have begun to give me discomfort so I am back on the pain patch. They will do a second round of radiation to the two spots on Wednesday. The radiation really zeros in on the tumors and is considered to be extremely effective. Some folks lovingly prayed for me after Sunday's service and a wonderful group of angels came today to also pray for me. I am in awe and humbled by all the prayers on my behalf. The words "All is well with my soul for my God is in control. I know not His plans for me but I know that He holds me in the palm of His hands." truly comforts me. And what a wonderful place to be! Several weeks after my back surgery just prior to Christmas, I was feeling very low. I answered a call from a telemarketer. I am not sure what she was selling or exactly how the conversation went. I had pretty much dismissed it. The next day I sat with Tony and Darcy in the palliative care center where my doctor passed the tissue box around as he spent forty minutes with us. I had forgotten how to laugh and weeping had taken a strong hold over my heart. My doctor wanted to start me on anti-depressants as well as pain meds. I agreed to the pain meds but wanted to hold off on the anti depressants. When we arrived back home Tony checked the voicemail and there was a message from my angel, the telemarketer from the day before. She simply said to read Revelations 21:4. "And God shall wipe away all tears from their eyes; and there shall be no more death, neither sorrow, nor crying, neither shall there be any more pain: for the former things are passed away."

Joy,
Carol

April 15, 2013

We are moving about twelve miles from UVA. Our house sold quickly, thank You, Jesus. We have found a new home but will have to reside in an apartment for two months while it is being completed. This is a good thing; first floor master suite, no garden to tend and half the size, with room still for our children to have their spaces when they are with us. In my downsizing mode I found this photo of Chris & Darcy. It makes me smile every time I look at it. Chris finishes up his film program in June and plans to look for work and stay in the NY area. Darcy is finishing her third year in nursing and is off to Mayo Clinic in Minnesota for a summer ten-week externship. Thank you for all your prayers regarding my health. The tumors in my pelvic bone were radiated and I experienced almost overnight relief. A suspicious growth on my scalp was biopsied and is the same cancer. But I just received great news. The MRI performed last week showed the tumor to be not invasive. I will meet w/a head surgeon to remove the complete tumor they biopsied but no bone invasion or other head tumors were seen!! Again thank You, God, for this wonderful news. Our move is going surprisingly well. Tony and I did experience some seller's remorse but God has given us a "paradigm shift" and we now see this as a new adventure! Praying you all see God at work in your lives and see all the blessings He bestows on each of us. God Bless.

Love,
Carol & family

May 18, 2013 - New Phase

Hi there CaringBridge World. This past week has been a rather eventful one in the Alimenti household. On Monday my mom had surgery to remove the tumor from her head and a skin graft was taken from her thigh to replace the skin removed from her head. Despite some rocky moments, overall the recovery has been going well. Yesterday and today my parents moved from their three-story home in Charlottesville to a temporary apartment in Crozet until their new home is completed in July (for move number two). Needless to say, it was quite the downsize. However, they have adjusted quite nicely to their quaint one-bedroom apartment and have nestled in next to the Blue Ridge Mountains. Thank you everyone for your support and prayers both with the move and the surgery. We are still waiting on the pathology report, and will hopefully know more when my mom goes to her doctor's appointment next week.

Love and Blessings,
Darcy
"Have I not commanded you? Be strong and courageous. Do not be frightened, and do not be dismayed, for the Lord your God is with you wherever you go." Joshua 1:9

July 22, 2013

We are settling into our new home nicely. It was a perfect move, we now have just enough space and we love the new area. Tony and I take long walks, ride our bikes, and admire the mountains and the spectacular sunsets. We feel like honeymooners. I feel so blessed to be here and have this time with Tony. Darcy is nearing the end of her summer in Minnesota. She has loved the learning experience as well as living in a new part of the country and meeting new folks. Chris finished his film certification program and is actively searching for employment. He lives in Harlem, five flights up, no elevator! I have been feeling great despite a not so great recent scan. They found two new liver lesions, one new paraspinal muscle lesion, and two new lesions in my lumbar. I have started a diet developed at Johns Hopkins for epilepsy patients, which is an extremely low carb diet. Some positive research w/mice and metastasis shrinking prompted me to give it a try. I will see how my September upper body and October lower body scans go. The theory is that cancer thrives on sugar, carbs turn into sugar, low carbs = starving cancer cells. Praying it does just that, **shrivel up all the tumors**! Won't that be something to shout about!!! Thank you for walking this journey with us. Your prayers matter. God is good.

Love and God bless,
Carol & family

October 1, 2013

I am still on my "starving cancer cell" diet. October 30th, the lower half of my body will be scanned. This will mark four months on the diet and four months since the last scan of this area. Stability even will be a big accomplishment. Not to be morbid but more to proclaim God's mercy, I recently counted my tumors, one primary, thirteen either radiated or cut out, and seventeen being observed. This November 20th will mark my five-year anniversary since diagnosis. Median survival is fifteen months! So God is good and He does answer our prayers. This weekend at a UVA pinning

166

ceremony for Darcy, the parents in front of us heard her name. They asked if I was Carol. Turns out for the last year they and their nursing student daughter have been praying for me daily. A long time ago I heard a quote, "The saddest day will be going to heaven and hearing about all the tears that were shed for all the prayers that were not prayed." I am forever grateful for all the prayers that have been and are being prayed in my name. It is so so humbling and so uplifting! Thank you all. On the home front, Darcy is in her last year, a busy, busy co-ed! Chris is working hard, making rent, living in NYC. Not an easy feat but he is happy with his independence and pursuit of his dreams. Tony is busy with work and caring for me! I have a wonderful palliative care team at UVA. They manage my symptoms and even started me on a low dose of Ritalin to give me a boost of energy. I go and then I rest and I repeat the cycle. I feel so blessed to have this time with family and friends. God is good. May you all experience His Joy, His Peace, and His Love.

God Bless,
Carol

November 4, 2013 - Surprise

As a young girl I would slyly unwrap the Christmas presents hidden in the eaves of the attic and carefully rewrap them so my snooping ways would go undetected. I also never liked roller coasters. I hated the adrenaline rush that comes with riding a roller coaster. I wanted to know what came next, no surprises. God has been teaching me, however, that life is full of surprises and more importantly, I need not fear them. My recent scan was just that, full of surprises. The cancer has become very aggressive, lots of growth and new sites. But here lies the good news, I no longer have to be the model patient, trying every possible alternative/ natural remedy. I can eat my dark chocolate and sip my wine without guilt. I will, with the Lord's help, allow the surprises, the mysteries of life to unfold one day at a time. My prayer is that with each new day I can remember to smile, to find things to be thankful for, to keep my head up, mindful of Jesus, to not miss an opportunity to give a compliment, to not forget to say I love you, and to keep my heart hopeful. And I am thankful to you for all the prayers you have sent up in my name.

Love and God Bless,
Carol

November 25, 2013 - Give Thanks

Today I completed round five of radiation to my hip. I am not new to this treatment; I know the staff, the equipment, the basic routine. But I am always amazed at how they change things based on what area of your body they are radiating. I have had a full body mask made, I have been wrapped in pink plastic and this time I was given circular, blue foam tube and was told to hold it and pretend I was driving a Ferrari. Another aspect of radiation involves music. During my initial experiences I was allowed to bring in CDs. More recently, they have created genres to choose from. For my Ferrari excursions I started w/a little Motown then mixed it up with some easy listening and classical pieces. Today it was all about Motown as I happily cruised in my imaginary sports car. But things quickly switched to our family friendly mini-van with two screeching teeny ones strapped into their car seats, with Tony at the wheel. Desperate parents, searching for calm, created the thank you game. Tony and I would start the ball rolling and within minutes smiles grew on all our faces and peace filled our van. Today I experienced the most emotional treatment I have received thus far. As I laid on the treatment table, tears streamed down my cheeks. Give thanks. Thank You, Lord, for a loving husband, two wonderful children, a devoted family, friends and church, nurses, doctors, technicians, available treatments, time to watch my children grow into adults and the prayers of so many. So much to give thanks for. Below are the lyrics that took over the Motown sounds today. Happy Thanksgiving.

Love and God bless,
Carol
"Give thanks with a grateful heart.
Give thanks unto the Holy One.
Give thanks because He's given Jesus Christ, His Son.

Give thanks with a grateful heart.
Give thanks unto the Holy One.
Give thanks because He's given Jesus Christ, His Son.
And now let the weak say, 'I am strong.'
Let the poor say, 'I am rich.'
Because of what the Lord has done for us.
And now let the weak say, 'I am strong.'
Let the poor say, 'I am rich.'
Because of what the Lord has done for us."
AMEN!

March 4, 2014 - Transitions

Early December, during my visit with my Palliative doctor, she said she would like to transition my care to Hospice. I defiantly replied, "I am going to my daughter's graduation in May!" Her response caused me some alarm. "If you begin to decline rapidly, have an early celebration. If you make it to her graduation, celebrate again." I needed time to process things. I wasn't ready for this next step. A few days later God gently whispered in my ear, "Celebrate each day." With God's assurance I was ready to transition to this next phase of care. On the heels of this news came the news that Chris needed to take a break from the stresses of NYC and was moving back to Virginia. We turned his move into a Big Apple holiday. Darcy joined us in the city, where we celebrated with friends and family, took in Broadway, and enjoyed life together. God so blessed Chris's decision that by January 1st he had a great rental, wonderful roommates in a fun section of Charlottesville, a job at a coffee house, and enrolled in school, determined to complete the remaining classes needed to get his associate's degree. We rang in the New Year in a highly festive fashion, we attended a masked gala ball at a local winery. We danced, laughed, and celebrated life. Hospice started after the New Year and has been such a gift. No more scans, tests, blood work, or treks to the hospital. I have a loving team weekly come to our home to check on me, pray with me, even my meds are delivered to my door. I am given time to build relationships with the individuals who will be caring for me in my final days.

Tony's mom has had a rough couple of years due to strokes and falls. Shortly after Christmas a stroke left her in the hospital. While they were trying to insert a port she suffered multiple cerebral strokes. She was transitioned to a hospice bed and passed ten days later, three days shy of her eighty-first birthday. Tony's dad, Carl, is now mourning the loss of his bride of nearly sixty years. We had a lovely memorial service last month celebrating her life.

To escape this cold winter, Tony and I headed to Florida. We sandwiched a cruise in between family visits. I didn't know a cruise was even on my bucket list but I am now glad I had the opportunity to check it off. We were blessed with no travel glitches, no health issues and eighty-degree sunshine every day. I set a goal to not take the elevator during the eight days at sea. I met my goal and also participated in a 5k cancer walk aboard ship. Not bad for a lady two months into hospice care! God is good. Darcy is in the final stretch at UVA. She is beginning the interviewing process. We pray that God will direct her to the place where He wants her to begin her career in nursing. It is an exciting and scary time for her but she will be a wonderful oncology nurse.

I am busy with a bucket list item, getting ready for an art exhibit of my work this spring. We are enjoying our new home. We, with the Lord's help, remain thankful as we celebrate life each day. It is a precious gift He bestows on us. I am thankful to you all for sharing in this gift of life.

Love and God bless,
Carol & family

November 20, 2014 - Thankful

Six years ago today I was told I had stage IV uterine leiomyosarcoma, an extremely rare cancer without a cure. Tomorrow marks eight years since Chris was told he had leukemia. We are so thankful for Chris remaining in remission and that I am here to celebrate yet another Thanksgiving with my family. God is good. I apologize for not updating you sooner. I am still on hospice, closing in on the end of eleven months, long past Darcy's graduation. She has now moved on to Johns Hopkins working in their stem cell transplant unit, helping very ill patients. But it is where her heart lies. Chris lives in Charlottesville, about a half hour from us. He is working and doing well. We get to see him often, so we are so thankful to have him here. We miss Darcy but she comes home often and we will all be together for Thanksgiving with my sister and her family in Annapolis. My health has shown a minimal decline over the last year. I have received radiation twice but all in all, not too bad. I paint and have even sold several paintings. I take art lessons, Tony and I both tutor at an after school program through our church, and I attend a ladies' Bible study, a church home group, all of which I love. I keep expecting hospice to kick me out but they have told me my diagnosis alone is enough to keep me in their services. They are a blessed group of people and I am so thankful to have them in my life, as I am all of you. So God bless you all and happy Thanksgiving.

Love,
Carol and family

May 31, 2015 - Update on Carol

Sorry as it has been a while. To start with, Carol has experienced a gradual decline that was most severe around Christmas time and has since stabilized. At present, she sleeps approximately three-fourths of the day with oxygen to assist with breathing. We have a walker in the wings, but she still has relative good stability. Her immune system has weakened and her latest battle is thrush. She has no real appetite. She has episodes of acute pain, which are managed with an array of drugs and we are thankful for the resources we have to control the pain. Hospice has been wonderful. Someone is here practically every day. As a result of the decline, visitors have come to totally stress and wear her out. Her best times are with both of her children by her side, which is the current situation. We are so thankful they are both at home. I'll try to be more vigilant on updates. Thank you for all your support, love, & prayers. We ask for continued prayer for peace, pain management, and strength.

Love,
Tony

June 24, 2015

As promised, here is my latest update on Carol's health status. The biggest hurdle is falling. Not that she fell (because we caught her) she can't even get out of bed without one of us helping her. I tease that I get to dance with her when we move from the bed to wherever. She will really miss her bi-weekly bath due to the fall risk. We have a shower seat that works perfectly and she loves it. She has been running periodic fevers and experiencing periodic states of confusion. She has had a choir of angels singing at her bedside, and one morning at 2 a.m. she requested a treat: a bagel with lox and cream cheese (fortunately Darcy had picked up the ingredients the day before). She sleeps until ~ 4 p.m. each day. We then move her over to the great room so she can have some social time. We have been enjoying the men's baseball CWS, which has kept her up cheering for UVA until 11 p.m. Thank you for all your prayers, and we send our love to each and every one of you.

Carol, Tony, Chris, and Darcy

July 8, 2015

Carol has been relatively stable lately. No major pain breakthroughs. She continues to run periodically a low temperature, which depletes what little energy she has. Physically she has been getting some small bruises, probably due to low platelets, her joints ache, and she has some redness on her palms, as well as periodic labored breathing and some recent coughing/choking. On occasions she has ventured out to our little courtyard, and cherishes time with her children.

July 22, 2015

Not much to say except we are seeing some symptoms of liver failure, as well as various bone and skin tumor pressure pain. We are thankful for the time we have with her and enjoying the opportunity for family togetherness, thank you for all your inquiries and prayers.

Love,
the Alimentis

August 20, 2015

Carol has been feeling more tired and experiencing more pain. The tumors are starting to become more visible on the outside. For example, the one on her back is fortunately growing outward instead of towards the spinal cord. It has the appearance of a large Idaho potato. Hospice has been working with different combinations of pain management modalities, being cognizant to minimize any negative side effects. One thing they are trying is to have her on steroids, which had one positive side effect of giving her more energy. This has enabled her to partake in some of her favorite activities. She has actually sketched a little and gotten into the courtyard to enjoy the garden and the hummingbirds. Thanks for your continued prayers and support.

Love,
the Alimentis

September 18, 2015

The song "Stairway to Heaven" comes to mind as I reflect on the last few weeks. My mother has climbed a new step on her journey towards eternity. She has reached a new level of weakness. The onset came on quickly and resulted in two falls leaving her with multiple bruises, scrapes, a black eye, and overall soreness. She can no longer walk on her own and now relies on a wheelchair and us for mobility. She has also had some periods of confusion. Pain continues to be an issue, however, we are learning how best to manage this symptom. Darcy resigned from her job in Baltimore and her family is experiencing the value of her four years of nursing education firsthand. Our family of four is now under one roof, uniting in care for our beloved Carol. We are all looking forward to Monday to celebrate Chris' twenty-fifth birthday. Despite the uncertainty and fear with this new step towards Heaven, the Lord remains our constant source of peace. Thank you for your prayers, love, & support.

Blessings,
the Alimentis

October 29, 2015

Over the last week Carol has spent most of her days asleep. We wake her to eat, but she often finds fatigue calling her to shut her eyes. She also has become too weak to walk at all. Thankfully, she has a strong and supportive husband to help her get to the bedside commode. Carol now uses the oxygen all the time to help with breathing as the ascites (fluid in her abdomen) made it harder for her to breath. With the addition of methadone to her already complex pain medication regimen, Carol has found relief. Positioning, however, has become key as Carol is now lovingly referred to as the "Princess and the Pea" atop her mountain of pillows, surrounded by her children and husband. Our only regret is that we don't have a king-size bed for us all to rest in. :) Dying is not easy, but supportive hospice workers, loving family, prayers from friends and family, and trust and hope in a Heaven without pain, suffering, and tears bring comfort. Thank you. God Bless. Happy Halloween.

The Alimentis.

December 5, 2015

Ann, Carol's mother, carried this quote in her purse: *Life should not be a journey to the grave with the intention of arriving safely in a pretty and well-preserved body, but rather to skid in broadside in a cloud of smoke, thoroughly used up, totally worn out and proclaiming "Holy Shit! What a ride!"* Carol's journey to the grave has been anything but easy. November marked seven years from her diagnosis with terminal cancer. Recently, Carol has been suffering from increased pain, restlessness, nausea, anxiety, delirium, hallucinations, and agitation. On Thursday night, after maxing out on all oral medication options, we took her to the emergency department. With hospice and palliative care's guidance, Carol now has a PICC line (central IV) allowing her to receive pain medication continuously. She is currently still at UVA Hospital as the teams try to develop a plan to manage her complex symptoms, so that Carol can return home and rest peacefully. Unfortunately, Carol still has a long road ahead of her and her symptoms will likely continue to worsen despite treatment. And so, I humbly come before you and ask you to please pray for my father, Chris, and myself, that we may have the strength and knowledge to care for our dear Carol. But most importantly we ask that you pray that the hospice and palliative care teams can help relieve Carol's suffering so that we can bring her back home and that she will be able to finish this journey to the grave as she intended: in her own bed, surrounded by loved ones, quietly, peacefully, and painlessly, in her sleep. Love and Gratitude.

Darcy

December 13, 2015 - "Rest Now, Dear Mommy"

At 7:55 a.m. my mommy passed the way she wanted: at home, in the arms of my daddy, surrounded by Chris and I, and as comfortable as earthly possible. My mother was the rock of our family, the source of love, the life of the party. She was the creator of beauty. Whether it be gardens, paintings, homes, or meals everything my mommy touched was transformed into a masterpiece. And though we miss her dearly and are now left with holes in our hearts, we find solace in knowing my mommy has been made whole. Her illness is no more, her pain and suffering complete, and her tears dried. Today my mother has been set free *"to dance with the angels on streets made of gold."* So grateful to call you my mommy, my friend, my kindred spirit. Rest now, dear mommy.
Rest in the arms of Our Savior.

Love you to the Moon and Back,
Darcy, Chris, & Tony

Memorial Service Messages

Song to Carol
by Chris Alimenti

All my memories of her drift,
but her spirit lives on
from the moon and the stars
to where the high-above clouds
lift.

Time rambles on
and the birds soar back
in the mist of Spring
as my past memories are gone.

I tremble at the pain
of all the loved ones lost.
Leaving me alone, to beg,
Oh God, who's gonna keep me
sane?

When I look up to the sky
everything seems to fly on by
like a flash in the wind.
When I look up to the sky.

As the wind roars
and the sun beams down
I can feel her spirit
knocking at my door.

She adored the children she bore
fighting for their lives
even in the days
of the cancer war.

In the deep of my soul
she lives on
in the trees, the wind, and rain.
Still fighting for our life's soul.

When I look up to the sky
everything seems to fly on by

like a flash in the wind.
When I look up to the sky.

When I look up to the sky.

Tribute to Carol
By Darcy Alimenti

Before I begin, I would like to thank each of you for your friendship, love, and support. My mother was a miraculous woman with an energy that attracted people and radiated love. Thank you for loving this woman so dear to my heart.

I titled my tribute to my mother "Lessons My Mommy Taught Me." Carol was not only my mother; she was my best friend, and my first and most influential teacher. Her life is a testimony of grace and hope despite suffering and loss. I would like to share with you some of the lessons that this remarkable lady I call Mom instilled in me:

The only way to have a friend is to be a friend.

During the last few months of my mother's life and after her passing, people — friends, neighbors, Hospice workers, relatives, etc. — referred to my mother as a "dear friend." They even joked that Carol had a way of making everyone feel like they were indeed her best friend. How could one person have such an impact on so many people? It was her love for people and relationships. My mom always said that we are here on Earth for relationships. She lived a life that reflected this value for people and for deep and meaningful connections. She always looked for those that looked lonely; she knew the exact questions to ask to get people to open up. She engaged fully with those she was with. She always could find a common subject to talk about with others — gardening, art, wine, travel, etc. She always saw the best in people and openly expressed the unique ways they were special.

Every good soup begins with a soffritto.

My mother was an amazing cook. It was one of the many

ways she shared her love for others. She could throw the contents of our fridge and pantry together and create a gourmet, delicious meal. She loved to host and break bread with friends and loved ones. Christmas Eve, field hockey, pasta nights, St. Patty's Day, picnics, and the ordinary weeknight meals were her way of sharing her love for food and embracing her Italian/Irish roots. Many of my memories take place around my family dining room table. She loved to plan meals days in advance. The moment we finished one meal, she was already creating and inquiring about our preferences for the next. One of the hardest losses my mother endured was the loss of energy she needed to be the gracious host and fine chef. This reality meant that my father and I were now the head chefs. My mother had to transition from the creator to the director. And despite some pretty thickheaded students, she graciously took on her new role as instructor. During her last year, my father, Chris, and I soaked up as many recipes and tips as we could from my mother. And here is a tidbit I shall share with you. Every good soup starts with a *soffritto* – olive oil, red pepper flakes, salt, pepper, minced celery, carrots, onion, and garlic. Sauté these ingredients until they are lightly browned, and you will have the savory base for most Italian soups.

Laughter is good for the heart.

When Chris got sick my mom, purchased him every season of *Everybody Loves Raymond* and *Seinfeld*. Laughter is how we would overcome. People often speak of my mom's glowing smile, but she also had a contagious laugh. In life's hardest moments, she always searched for ways to bring life and laughter. At a young age, her Aunt Vera nicknamed her "the Joker." I loved hearing stories of how, when they were growing up, she and her dear friend Laurie used to put on performances and musicals for the family. She could perform "If I Were a Rich Man" from *Fiddler on the Roof* like the original Tevye. She would drop everything to join me in performing "Second Hand Rose" from *Funny Girl*. She had such a positive energy that always filled the room.

It's not just a religion, it's a relationship.

Mom lived with constant pain. The large number of tumors she had scattered throughout her body made it difficult to manage her pain. A warm bath, however, was one way she found relief. She loved her bath time. She would light candles and play music from her iPod and soak for hours. I used to tease her that she would turn into a prune. One day, I went to check on her when I heard some noises. As I entered the bathroom, I heard her talking to God as if she were conversing with my dad or Chris, confiding in Him her fears of pain, and dying, and leaving loved ones. It turned out that these sacred bath times were so special to my mother because they were, more importantly, prayer times. Time when she could find comfort and focus on her Savior, her Father, her source of strength, hope, joy, and life. When my mom became too weak for baths and too tired to formulate the words, she and my father took on a nightly ritual of reciting the Lord's Prayer, the Hail Mary, and Psalm 23. My mom's faith and trust and hope despite such trying times were and are such a testimony to those of us that knew her.

Life's too short to not take trips.

Shortly after my mom's diagnosis with cancer, she decided that vacations should be a priority. And so, bald, fluid-overloaded, and a week after failing chemotherapy, my mother boarded a flight to France with my family. Our tour of France's countryside marked the beginning of many amazing trips my family took together. After our second international vacation, my father teased that we would go broke from our extravagant vacations as my mother lived to one hundred years old, all the while crossing trip after trip off of her bucket list. To which my mother replied, "Tony, think of all the beautiful places we will see and the memories we will make." And that statement depicts so perfectly my mother's desire: to make sweet memories with those she loved.

Follow your heart.

My mother loved art. Throughout her life, she found ways to make art a part of her routine. She took art classes as a young adult with my grandmother; pottery classes with me as a child, and, after Chris and I graduated high school, she began taking art classes at Piedmont Community College. Mind you, she was three years into her cancer diagnosis at this point in her life. She loved drawing, sketching, and painting. She dreamed of becoming an art teacher at one of the local high schools. And she even wanted to have an art show — it was on her bucket list. Well, let me tell you, where there's a will, there's a way. And Carol followed her heart and ended up having two art shows, and even sold a total of five paintings. Her life is the quintessential example of resilience.

These are only a few of the many lessons my mother taught me. My heart aches, as her loss has left a large void in my life. However, my mother didn't believe in goodbyes; it always had to be "See you later." And so, Mom, this isn't goodbye. This is "see you later." Thank you for the love, joy, and hope with which you surrounded me. I am so grateful to be called Carol's daughter, and I look forward to the day I can hold you again in the House of the Lord. See you later, Mom. Love, your Darcy.

Tribute to Carol

By Tony Alimenti

Thank you all for coming. It is such a blessing to us and to Carol, and I'd like to thank the church, and my home group, for making this memorial service happen.

We all have known or been touched by Carol in different ways. I tried to keep this to ten minutes, but found that I couldn't. Every time I'd try to summarize my time with Carol, I'd remember another story or adventure. There are thousands of these adventures, stories, memories, and laughs I could share. Even five hours would not be enough time.

Maybe I can hit some highlights (each with its own story around the adventure). I'd love to share and laugh over our individual stories sometime.

Carol and I first caught each others' eye twenty-eight years ago, from across the room at a "yuppy" happy hour in NJ. The rest is history. "She had me..."

I was taken away in the surging river that was Carol. We talked — or, should I say: she talked, and I listened, enamored — about hiking, step vans, California, UC Berkeley, wineries...

As time went on, and knowing Carol as we all did, I'm sure you can guess that our favorite topics included entertaining, outdoor activities, gardening, painting, decorating, house renovations, bargain hunting...and a few more I'm sure I'm missing. These all may appear different, but from Carol's perspective, they were all an artist's palette of life. She did and approached everything with a passion. There was always a home or landscape to critique or enhance. We never passed up visiting a local garden or garden tour — after which we would go home and promptly try implementing what we had seen. She was a Virginia Tech Certified Master Gardener.

"The garden path should weave," she would say, "so that you are forced to divert your view so as to enjoy the walk, see and smell the flowers, and sit on a bench and take in the beauty."

She loved decorating. She would scour magazines for decorating ideas and somehow implement them without breaking the bank. A true bargain hunter, she quickly found every thrift and consignment shop wherever we were. No discarded roadside furniture pile went un-investigated.

Carol loved the challenge of tweaking décor, furniture arrangements, and picture and flower placements. She had a business called "Heavenly Habitats," and always worked toward making our own habitats heavenly.

She painted walls, tiles, and canvases; met her goal of selling a few paintings; and even got a commissioned job! She worked in PR for a couple of wineries, and was a VP of Sales at a number of different technical headhunter agencies. She dabbled in real estate. She became an excellent caregiver and advocate: first for her kids; then her mother; and finally, for herself.

She was an expert in reading and interpreting CBC and liver panel reports, as well as CT, MRI, and PET scans. She would scour the internet and the NIH for the latest on potential cures, clinical studies, and treatment options. She would research various foods, supplements, and exercises — anything that would better the chances of survival for herself or one of her family members. She became an expert in the three A's: antioxidants, anti-inflamatories, antiangiogenics. That's probably why she fought and lived so fully and successfully for seven years with a cancer that has an average survival rate of fifteen months! After each surgery, radiation, or chemo treatment, she would bounce back. She was fighting to be in life.

She would walk, swim, bike, yoga, and just "come back" to be a part of life, to embrace the next new reality. Books, crosswords, puzzles, Sudoku, board and card games from Farkle to Scrabble, thumbing through magazines...these were her indulgences. I knew she wasn't feeling well when she would only beat me by fifty points in Scrabble!

Even in the midst of battling cancer, she orchestrated

183

vacations and family outings. She took us to France, Ireland, Italy, Colorado, Arizona, and the Caribbean. We went on garden and house tours, on hot-air balloon rides, and attended social events from weddings to wine pairings to dancing.

She always had an eye toward enjoying life's gifts. She would create elegant fine dining or intimate gatherings with friends, and feasts or cookouts for friends and family, including some wonderful and amazing holiday events...any reason to celebrate together.

Then there were the birthday parties for the kids. Now, these weren't your normal birthday parties. They were elaborate topical events. Snow White-themed parties with painted castles on the basement walls, Peter Pan parties with zip lines, cakes baked into characters, stations for making coiled pots, capes for superhero adventures...

Even our daily meals had what I call a "Carol flair" to them. They were not only healthy, but had all the food groups, and were color coordinated. And of course, the elegant place setting and flower bouquet.

Always the host, she had hospitality in her blood. She loved people and building good relationships. Any room she walked into she'd meet and make friends, greeting all with a smile and a warmth that would melt you.

Beyond participating in various types of Bible studies over the years, she would have verses and sayings taped around the house to uplift our spirits, or help us focus on the important things in life. She loved being a greeter at church. That way, she could get to know everybody and be part of their story. She was an organizer, a tutor, and a volunteer on mission trips and in service events.

In all, she just loved being a part of what life offered. She planted many gardens and flowers in her life, both literally and figuratively. She tried to make the best of any situation, and tried to bring beauty and love to each encounter. She had a little plaque that stated: "A life without friends is like a garden without flowers." Whether it be a garden, a house, or a friend, whatever plot was set before her, she tried to build something on it and add a little beauty to it. These two verses come to mind when I think of Carol:

Ecclesiastes 3:12,13: "...there is nothing better for people than to be happy and to enjoy themselves as long as they live, and that everyone should eat and drink and find enjoyment in all their toil, for these things are a gift from God."

And Ecclesiastes 12:13: "...love God and love your neighbor."

You all are a wonderful garden and tribute to the love she spread and left in the hearts of all of us. I thank God for allowing me to walk with Carol in this life, if even for a little while.

Carol, it has been a real pleasure living life with you, planting so many gardens and enjoying the fruits of our toil—all the friends, food, memories, and adventures together...

I love you. Rest in peace, finally pain free, enjoying the next garden you are tending in Heaven.

Thank you, and God bless you.

December 16, 2015

Carol Alimenti, 62, of Charlottesville, departed her earthly habitat to meet her Savior the morning of December 13, 2015. Carol passed peacefully in her home seven years after her diagnosis of uterine leiomyosarcoma (ULMS) cancer, surrounded by her loving husband and children. She is survived by her husband (Anthony), two children (Christopher and Darcy), her siblings (Anne, Michael, and Joyce), as well as many cousins, nieces, nephews, aunts, uncles, and friends. Carol took life's challenges in stride. Carol, the poster child for ULMS, also idealized the concept of dying with dignity as a patient of palliative care for a year and hospice care for two years. She was an engaging conversationalist, with a radiating smile, a gift for hospitality, and an eye for enhancing the palette of life before her. She was the creator of beauty. Whether it be serene gardens, exquisite paintings, elegant homes, or gourmet meals, everything Carol touched was transformed into a masterpiece. She was an amazing spirit who loved and lived life with a passion for people and relationships. She touched the hearts of many, and those she left behind will be forever changed.

A Memorial Service to honor Carol's precious life will take place on January 9th at 11:00 a.m. at Christ Community Church, with a reception to follow.

Donations may be made in Carol's memory to:

- UVA School of Nursing: www.nursing.virginia.edu UVA
- Emily Couric Cancer Center: www.uvahealth.com
- Hospice of Piedmont: www.hopva.org

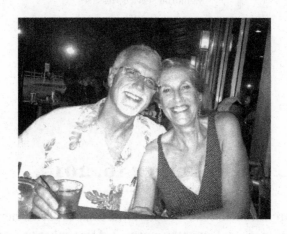

Carol Alimenti

Carol, a New Jersey native, was drawn to the Blue Ridge Mountains of Charlottesville, Virginia, in 2004 with her husband, Tony, and their two children, Christopher and Darcy. An environmental science graduate from UC Berkeley, Carol was also a painter, chef, Master Gardener, lover of the outdoors, and designer of gardens and interior spaces. She had a passion for the arts, and for finding and creating beauty in life. *My Turn on the Couch* is Carol's first and only book. She passed away in 2015.

Anthony Alimenti

Anthony Charles Alimenti, nicknamed Tony — or as his wife Carol called him, "Ant-ny" — worked for over thirty years as an engineer in the telecommunications industry. He met his wife Carol while they lived in New Jersey, where they had two kids: Darcy and Christopher. He was a caregiver with Carol; first for their son when he battled cancer, and then for Carol's mother, until she passed while living with them. Then he and his children provided care for Carol through seven years of her battle with cancer.

Anthony recently retired to Crozet, Virginia, where he spends his time participating in various men's groups, playing guitar, golfing, and trying to learn Italian.

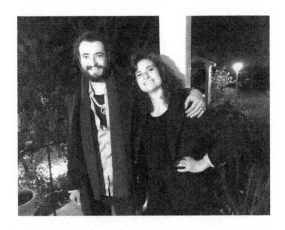

Chris Alimenti

Chris Alimenti was born in Little Silver, New Jersey, and lived there until 2004 with his sister, Darcy, his mother, Carol, and his father, Anthony. Chris suffered from seizures and earaches as a young child, which may have caused his audio-processing disorder. He learns in a hands-on and visual style, which prompted the family move to Charlottesville, Virginia for better school systems and, of course, for the Blue Ridge Mountains. Chris attended Murray High School, a charter school that focuses on kids who learn in a different, more abstract manner. At the age of sixteen, while attending Murray High School, he was diagnosed with Acute Lymphatic Leukemia (ALL), a blood cancer. Two years from the day of his diagnosis, his mother was diagnosed with uterine-based leiomyosarcoma (ULMS).

Chris is a cancer survivor, and recently completed a camping trip around the United States. He currently lives in Richmond, Virginia, attending Virginia Commonwealth University as an English major.

Darcy Alimenti

Darcy Alimenti, daughter of Carol and Anthony Alimenti, was thrust into the nursing profession at the mere age of fourteen as she cared for her brother, mother, and grandmother. After completing her formal nursing education at the University of Virginia School of Nursing, she worked as a registered nurse on an adult bone marrow transplant unit and an adult intensive care unit. She has stepped away from bedside nursing to pursue educational opportunities at the University of Pennsylvania School of Nursing, where she is studying to be an acute care gerontology nurse practitioner with a specialty in palliative care. In caring for her dying mother, Darcy developed a passion for holistic nursing that preserves the dignity of the dying and focuses on healing the soul. Darcy's goal in life is to embody the beauty, joy, love, and genuine nature of her late friend, role model, confidante: her mother.

CPSIA information can be obtained
at www.ICGtesting.com
Printed in the USA
BVOW03s1825250717
489998BV00001B/1/P